Topics in Neuroscience

M. Filippi • G. Comi • M. Rovaris (Eds)

Normal-appearing White and Grey Matter Damage in Multiple Sclerosis

Springer

Massimo Filippi
Neuroimaging Research Unit
Department of Neuroscience
Scientific Institute and University
Ospedale San Raffaele, Milan, Italy

Giancarlo Comi
Department of Neurology
Scientific Institute and University
Ospedale San Raffaele, Milan, Italy

Marco Rovaris
Neuroimaging Research Unit
Department of Neuroscience
Scientific Institute and University
Ospedale San Raffaele, Milan, Italy

The Editors and Authors wish to thank SCHERING S.p.A. for the support and help in the realization and promotion of this volume

---

Library of Congress Cataloging-in-Publication Data: Applied for

ISBN 978-88-470-2175-4 ISBN 978-88-470-2127-3 (eBook)
DOI 10.1007/978-88-470-2127-3

springeronline.com

Originally published by Springer Milan Berlin Heidelberg New York in 2004

Typesetting: Color Point Srl (Milan)

Cover design: Simona Colombo

Introduction

M. Filippi, M. Rovaris, G. Comi

The pathological process of multiple sclerosis (MS) leads to the formation of macroscopic discrete foci of tissue damage in the central nervous system (CNS). These lesions can be seen on conventional magnetic resonance imaging (MRI) scans, making conventional MRI an extremely sensitive tool with which to diagnose MS and monitor its evolution. Nevertheless, there are discrepancies between the clinical and the neuroradiological aspects of MS: MRI-visible damage is not sufficient to explain the entire spectrum of manifestation of the disease.

There is a growing body of evidence that MS pathology does not spare the normal-appearing white (NAWM) and grey (NAGM) matter, since a wide range of abnormalities are detectable outside MS lesions using either histopathological or MRI techniques. Such changes may be either secondary to intrinsic damage of lesions visible on T_2-weighted MRI, via wallerian degeneration of fibres passing through macroscopic abnormalities, or they may be the result of an independent pathological process affecting the normal-appearing tissues. In the NAWM, the main pathological findings are gliosis, microglial activation, disturbances of the blood-brain barrier and loss of axons. In the NAGM, less inflammatory changes are seen, but numerous lesions can be identified ex vivo which are not detectable on T_2-weighted MRI. In the last few years, the hypothesis that the accumulation of NAWM and NAGM damage may contribute to the progression of MS-related neurological disability has led to the challenge of quantifying in vivo the extent of such damage and to define the patterns of its changes over time. In this context, several MR-based techniques have been interrogated as tools able to provide reliable information about the heterogeneous aspects of NAWM and NAGM pathology of MS.

MR-based measurements of white and grey matter volumes represent a preliminary but useful tool to assess the final outcome of NAWM and NAGM damage, i.e. the occurrence and progression of tissue atrophy. The poor correlation between atrophy and T_2-visible lesion load, consistently reported by several studies of MS, supports the notion that white and grey matter volume reductions may primarily reflect MRI-occult pathology.

Among the more sophisticated and modern MR-based methodologies, magnetization transfer (MT) MRI is now widely applied in the study of MS, and the results of preliminary studies with this technique have provided the earliest in vivo evidence of NAWM and NAGM damage in MS. All these studies analysed the MT ratio (MTR) as a measure of the magnetization exchange between free and bound protons, whose decrease reflects a loss of the latter compartment. Correlative studies have confirmed that a significant relationship exists between decreased MTR and increased loss of myelin and axons, both within MS lesions and in the NAWM, and that NAWM MTR changes may precede the formation of new, MRI-visible lesions. Moreover, reduced NAWM MTR has been found to increase with increasing disease duration and disability. More recent data indicate that a similar MTR decrease can also be found in the NAGM from the earliest and non-disabling phases of MS.

The measurement of T_1 and T_2 relaxation characteristics may also enable us to detect subtle changes of tissue microstructure. The recent availability of 3-T magnets has made it possible to obtain whole-brain quantitative T1 maps in a few minutes, whereas it remains challenging to obtain T_2 decay curves from large portions of the brain. Both histogram analysis of T_1-relaxation times and evaluation of T_2 decay curves in the NAWM of MS patients indicate that myelin loss is the dominant pathological process in this tissue compartment. Preliminary studies have also interrogated T_1-relaxation time changes following gadolinium injection as a measure of subtle blood-brain barrier permeability breakdown in the NAWM, with the aim of achieving a more complete assessment of the MS-related inflammatory processes. Interestingly, other preliminary data seem to indicate a decrease of T_1-relaxation times in the NAGM, which may reflect pathological processes other than loss of myelin and axons, such as the deposition of iron accompanying neurodegeneration.

Diffusion-weighted imaging (DWI) is sensitive to the microscopic random motion of water molecules, which is the result of the interactions with structural barriers that can restrict it. Using DWI, the brain tissue microstructure can be interrogated, by means of quantitative indices such as the mean diffusivity (MD), which is a measure of the average molecular motion and is affected by cellular size and integrity, and fractional anisotropy (FA), which reflects the degree of alignment of cellular structures within fibre tracts, as well as their structural integrity. In MS patients, several studies have found significantly increased MD values and reduced FA values in the NAWM and NAGM. Since "inflammatory" changes and gliosis can potentially restrict water molecular motion, myelin and axonal damage appear to be the most likely contributors to the loss of barriers limiting water motion (increased MD) and to tissue structural organization (decreased FA). The recent development of DWI tractography offers a promising tool for exploring the involvement of clinically eloquent pathways in the NAWM of MS patients, as well as its relationship with concomitant grey matter damage and cortical functional changes.

Magnetic resonance spectroscopy (MRS) has the unique advantage of providing information with a high biochemical specificity for ongoing tissue changes. Single-voxel MRS and spectroscopic imaging data suggest that both inflammation and loss of axons contribute to NAWM pathology in MS, whereas the latter is largely predominant in the pathogenesis of NAGM damage. Longitudinal MRS studies have also provided evidence that NAWM pathology can be at least partially reversible when related to sub-lethal axonal damage of fibres crossing newly formed MS lesions.

The information provided by structural MR-based techniques about NAWM and NAGM damage in MS can be integrated with the data coming from functional MRI (fMRI) studies. This technique allows the ability of the MS brain to limit the consequences of irreversible tissue damage to be explored. fMRI data indicate that cortical reorganization in MS patients begins soon after the clinical onset of the disease and continues through the entire course of the disease. The extent of cortical reorganization has been found to correlate with the severity of NAWM and NAGM damage, as quantified by MTI, DWI, and MRS. All of this suggests that the rate of disability progression in MS might not only be a function of irreversible tissue damage, but also of the failure of cortical adaptive capacities.

Although new imaging modalities are needed that provide more specific in vivo measures of the various components of NAWM and NAGM pathology in MS, the contributions given by currently available structural and functional MR-based techniques are likely to be already valuable for monitoring the natural history of MS and its modification by treatment. In this book, we aim to provide an extensive summary of the state of the art and set the scenario for future research in the field of NAWM and NAGM damage in MS. We hope that the book will be of help to clinical neurologists and researchers, not only by allowing them to go deeper into this complex issue, but also by stimulating new ideas and further investigations.

Table of Contents

Normal-Appearing Grey Matter

List of Contributors

Arnold D.L.
Magnetic Resonance Spectroscopy Unit, Montreal Neurological Institute, McGill University, Montreal, Quebec, Canada

Bö L.
Department of Pathology, MS Center, VU University Medical Center, Amsterdam, The Netherlands. National Competence Center for MS, Department of Neurology, Haukeland University Hospital, Bergen, Norway

Brink B.P.
Department of Pathology, MS Center, VU University Medical Center, Amsterdam, The Netherlands

Brück W.
Department of Neuropathology, Georg-August University, Göttingen, Germany

Clare S.
Centre for Functional Magnetic Resonance Imaging of the Brain, Department of Clinical Neurology, University of Oxford, UK

Comi G.
Multiple Sclerosis Centre, Department of Neurology, Scientific Institute and University, Ospedale San Raffaele, Milan, Italy

De Stefano N.
Department of Neurological and Behavioral Sciences
Siena, Italy

Enzinger C.
Department of Neurology, Medical University Graz, Austria

Fazekas F.
Departments of Neurology and Neuroradiology, Medical University Graz, Austria

Filippi M.
Neuroimaging Research Unit, Department of Neurology, Scientific Institute and University
Ospedale San Raffaele, Milan, Italy

Gonen O.
Department of Radiology, New York University School of Medicine, New York, USA

Grossman R.I.
Department of Radiology, New York University School of Medicine, New York, USA

Inglese M.
Department of Radiology, New York University School of Medicine, New York, USA

Laule C.
Department of Physics and Astronomy, University of British Columbia, Vancouver, British Columbia, Canada

Li D.
Department of Radiology, University of British Columbia, Vancouver, British Columbia, Canada

MacInnes M.
Magnetic Resonance Spectroscopy Unit, Montreal Neurological Institute, McGill University, Montreal, Quebec, Canada

Mädler B.
Philips Medical Systems, Vancouver, British Columbia, Canada

MacKay A.
Departments of Physics and Astronomy and Radiology, University of British Columbia, Vancouver, British Columbia, Canada

Matthews P.M.
Centre for Functional Magnetic Resonance Imaging of the Brain, Department of Clinical Neurology, University of Oxford, UK

Miller D.H.
NMR Unit, Institute of Neurology, Queen Square, London, UK

Moore W.
Department of Pathology, University of British Columbia, Vancouver, British Columbia, Canada

Mörk S.J.
Department of Pathology, Haukeland University Hospital, Bergen, Norway

Parry A.M.
Centre for Functional Magnetic Resonance Imaging of the Brain, Department of Clinical Neurology, University of Oxford, UK

Paty D.
Department of Neurology, University of British Columbia, Vancouver, British Columbia, Canada

Rocca M.A.
Neuroimaging Research Unit, Department of Neurology, Scientific Institute and University Ospedale San Raffaele, Milan, Italy

Ropele S.
Departments of Neurology and Neuroradiology, Medical University Graz, Austria

Rovaris M.
Neuroimaging Research Unit, Department of Neurology, Scientific Institute and University Ospedale San Raffaele, Milan, Italy

Smith S.
Centre for Functional Magnetic Resonance Imaging of the Brain, Department of Clinical Neurology, University of Oxford, UK

Soon D.
NMR Unit, Institute of Neurology, Queen Square, London, UK

Stadelmann C.
Department of Neuropathology, Georg-August University, Göttingen, Germany

Traboulsee A.
Department of Neurology, University of British Columbia, Vancouver, British Columbia, Canada

van der Valk P.
Department of Pathology, MS Center, VU University Medical Center, Amsterdam, The Netherlands

Vavasour I.
Department of Radiology, University of British Columbia, Vancouver, British Columbia, Canada

Wegner C.
Centre for Functional Magnetic Resonance Imaging of the Brain, Department of Clinical Neurology, University of Oxford, UK

NORMAL-APPEARING WHITE MATTER

Chapter 1

Pathology of the Normal-Appearing White Matter in Multiple Sclerosis

W. Brück, C. Stadelmann

Introduction

Multiple sclerosis (MS) is regarded a chronic inflammatory disease of the central nervous system (CNS) leading to multifocal demyelinated plaques. The pathological hallmarks of the lesions are (1) inflammation with a cellular infiltrate consisting of T cells, a few B cells and macrophages/microglia; (2) demyelination with loss of oligodendrocytes in the chronic disease stage and a variable degree of remyelination especially in the early disease course; (3) axonal damage with significant axonal loss in chronic MS plaques; and (4) gliosis with astrocyte proliferation and intensive glial fibre production [1, 2]. The majority of MS patients start with a relapsing-remitting course, in which the inflammatory-demyelinating component of the disease predominates. In the progressive disease stage, which may be either primary or secondary, an additional neurodegenerative component appears to be involved [3], leading to extensive neuroaxonal damage in the chronic MS brain [4]. Loss of axons seems to be the major determinant of the persistent neurological deficit in the progressive disease stage of MS patients [5].

Pathological Characteristics of the MS Plaque

The characteristic features of an MS lesion are demyelinated plaques in the white matter of the CNS with relative axonal sparing and extensive glial scar formation [1]. Remyelination may also be present in MS lesions, especially in early disease phases [6]; its prevalence, however, may be underestimated due to the lack of remyelination-specific signals in magnetic resonance imaging (MRI) [7]. It is now widely accepted that the structural and immunopathological features of MS plaques are extremely variable, and that the events in MS immunopathogenesis may be more complicated than a pure T-cell-mediated autoimmune process leading to secondary macrophage activation and attack of the myelin sheath [8-12]. Oligodendrocytes and the myelin sheath seem to be the major target of the autoimmune response in MS. Oligodendrocytes are lost in the chronic disease stage. These cells are susceptible to damage by a broad panel of immunological or toxic effectors, including cytokines [13], reactive oxygen or nitrogen species, excitatory amino acids such as glutamate [14], complement components, proteolytic and lipolytic enzymes, T-cell-mediated injury via T-cell products (perforin/lymphotoxin) [15], the interaction of Fas antigen with Fas ligand [16], interaction of TRAIL (TNF-related apoptosis-related ligand) with its receptor [17], CD8+ class I MHC-mediated cytotoxicity [18], and persistent viral infection [19]. Proliferation of oligodendrocyte precursor cells with subsequent new formation of myelin sheaths – a process called remyelination – is frequently observed, mainly during the early stages of MS lesion formation [20, 21]. Remyelination clearly depends on the presence of oligodendrocytes within the lesion [22-24], and systematic studies on large MS tissue samples suggested that the fate of oligodendrocytes is extremely variable when lesions are compared between patients [12, 25].

All of these data suggest an interindividual heterogeneity of the pathogenetic mechanisms that lead to plaque formation in MS patients. This hypothesis was confirmed in recent studies showing that the pathogenic events involved in different subtypes of MS may be heterogeneous [10, 12]. Both the inflammatory infiltrates (T cells, B cells, macrophages/microglia) and the immunological effector molecules (antibody, complement, cytokines) present within the lesions show significant variations between individual MS patients. These observations suggest that different pathogenic mechanisms of demyelination may operate in different subgroups of MS patients.

MS is generally considered an inflammatory demyelinating disease of the CNS with relative axonal sparing. The pathology of axons in neurodegenerative or neuroinflammatory diseases may include loss, transection, or disturbed axonal transport. All these phenomena have already been long recognized in MS pathology [26]. In chronic MS lesions, there is a significant axonal loss of about 60% [27, 28]. However, acute axonal damage is also a characteristic sign of lesions formed in the early disease course [29]. All of these pathological changes in MS plaques may either be preceded by events occurring in the normal-appearing white matter (NAWM) or may have secondary effects on otherwise normal CNS tissue. These changes will be summarized in the following sections.

Normal-Appearing White Matter in MS

The basic paper on the pathology of the NAWM in MS was published by Allen and McKeown [30]. These authors combined histological, biochemical, and histochemical methods and found 72% of NAWM samples in MS patients to be abnormal. The definition of NAWM in this manuscript was "as far distant as possible from visible plaques". This macroscopic pathological definition may be different from that used in MRI studies. The main findings by Allen and McKeown were: (1) gliosis in 59.3% of the samples, (2) inflammation with the presence of small round cells (9.3%) or macrophages (13%), (3) perivascular deposits of lipofuscin (29.6%), (4) occasional unsuspected demyelination (13%), and (5) thickened blood vessels (5.6%). Additionally, they observed a significant increase in the lysosomal enzyme β-glucosaminidase. This increase was combined with a higher number of acid-phosphatase-positive cells. These observations, in summary, suggested that increased gliosis, a certain degree of macrophage/microglia activation, and sparse inflammation were the histological correlates of the NAWM pathology. The increased gliosis correlated with increased choline in MS NAWM as measured by magnetic resonance spectroscopy [31]. The morphological data were confirmed in a follow-up study, in which NAWM was defined as macroscopically normal tissue at least 1 cm distant from visible plaques [32]. Microglial activation in the NAWM was demonstrated by increased HLA-DR expression in this study and reduced myelin density was observed in conventional myelin stains. The different features of NAWM pathology will now be discussed in detail.

Inflammation and Blood-Brain Barrier Damage in the NAWM

Small round cell infiltrates, macrophages and microglial activation have been described initially as the main features of MS NAWM pathology [32]. Several recent papers focused on the presence of inflammatory mediators in MS lesions and the NAWM. Gobin et al. [33] found an upregulation of transcription factors controlling MHC expression by microglial cells. These cells were clustered in the NAWM to form nodule-type cell accumulations. Perivascular inflammatory infiltrates were also found in another study [34]. These cells were positive for molecules of the plasminogen activator and matrix metalloprotease cascade. Similar data were obtained in a parallel study mainly focusing on expression of matrix metalloproteinases and their inhibitors [35]. These molecules might lead to degradation of the extracellular matrix and thus facilitate entry of inflammatory cells into the CNS. One major function could also be the breakdown of the blood-brain barrier. Abnormal endothelial tight junctions were found in 15% of the blood vessels in the NAWM compared to 40% in MS lesions and <2% in normal controls [36]. These changes were observed in vessels of all calibres and were associated with fibrinogen leakage [37]. These data indicate that there are subtle changes at the blood-brain barrier in NAWM in MS, leading to leakage of serum proteins and allowing peripheral immune cells to enter the nervous system.

Axonal Pathology in the NAWM

There is clear evidence that axons are lost in MS plaques [27, 28] and that axonal transections are present in MS lesions [38, 39]. The distal part of a transected axon undergoes Wallerian degeneration [40] and is removed by microglia/macrophages [41]. If there is axonal loss in the NAWM, part of it could be explained by axonal pathology occurring in the lesions and subsequent Wallerian degeneration in the surrounding NAWM. These phenomena have convincingly been demonstrated by Bjartmar et al. [42] in a patient with acute MS. Other studies detected a significant axonal loss in MS NAWM with a reduction of axonal density and area [43]. In the corpus callosum, this regional axonal loss correlated with the lesion volume and distribution in the cerebral hemispheres [44]. Mainly small nerve fibres seem to be lost in the NAWM, and this loss can be observed from the early course of the disease onwards [45]. In addition, an abnormal ubiquitination of axons in the NAWM suggested a derangement of the proteolytic cascade in MS NAWM [46]. Magnetic resonance spectroscopy of MS patients revealed similar observations in the NAWM relating to axonal damage and Wallerian degeneration [47, 48].

Myelin/Oligodendrocyte Changes in the NAWM

There is one study describing selective loss of myelin-associated glycoprotein compared to other myelin proteins in the NAWM [49]. This observation might be linked to a certain subtype of MS pathology [10]. Oligodendrocyte survival factors such as insulin-like growth factor-I were not altered in MS NAWM [50]. These data suggest that myelin/oligodendrocytes are not the main focus of NAWM pathology.

Conclusions

The NAWM of MS patients is clearly altered and these changes can be observed pathologically and radiologically. The main pathological findings are: (1) gliosis, (2), perivascular inflammatory infiltration and microglial activation, (3) disturbances of the blood-brain barrier, and (4) loss of axons. Whether these changes represent a distinct and separate pathology of the NAWM in MS or whether these observations are secondary to the pathology of the demyelinating lesions remains to be clarified.

References

1. Lassmann H (1998) Pathology of multiple sclerosis. In: Compston A, Ebers G, Lassmann H et al (eds) McAlpine's multiple sclerosis. Churchill Livingstone, London, pp 323-358
2. Prineas JW (1985) The neuropathology of multiple sclerosis. In: Koetsier JC (ed) Demyelinating diseases. Elsevier Science, Amsterdam, pp 213-257
3. Lublin FD, Reingold SC (1996) Defining the clinical course of multiple sclerosis: results of an international survey. Neurology 46:907-911
4. Lassmann H (2003) Axonal injury in multiple sclerosis. J Neurol Neurosurg Psychiatry 74:695-697
5. Trapp BD, Ransohoff R, Rudick R (1999) Axonal pathology in multiple sclerosis: relationship to neurologic disability. Curr Opin Neurol 12:295-302
6. Brück W, Kuhlmann T, Stadelmann C (2003) Remyelination in multiple sclerosis. J Neurol Sci 206:181-185
7. Barkhof F, Brück W, De Groot CJ et al (2003) Remyelinated lesions in multiple sclerosis: magnetic resonance image appearance. Arch Neurol 60:1073-1081

8. Brück W, Lucchinetti C, Lassmann H (2002) The pathology of primary progressive multiple sclerosis. Mult Scler 8:93-97
9. Lassmann H, Brück W, Lucchinetti C (2001) Heterogeneity of multiple sclerosis pathogenesis: implications for diagnosis and therapy. Trends Mol Med 7:115-121
10. Lucchinetti C, Brück W, Parisi J et al (2000) Heterogeneity of multiple sclerosis lesions: implications for the pathogenesis of demyelination. Ann Neurol 47:707-717
11. Bitsch A, Brück W (2002) Differentiation of multiple sclerosis subtypes: implications for treatment. CNS Drugs 16:405-418
12. Lucchinetti C, Brück W, Parisi J et al (1999) A quantitative analysis of oligodendrocytes in multiple sclerosis lesions. A study of 113 cases. Brain 122:2279-2295
13. Bitsch A, Kuhlmann T, da Costa C et al (2000) Tumour necrosis factor alpha mRNA expression in early multiple sclerosis lesions: correlation with demyelinating activity and oligodendrocyte pathology. Glia 29:366-375
14. Pitt D, Nagelmeier IE, Wilson HC, Raine CS (2003) Glutamate uptake by oligodendrocytes: implications for excitotoxicity in multiple sclerosis. Neurology 61:1113-1120
15. Selmaj K, Cross AH, Farooq M et al (1991) Non-specific oligodendrocyte cytotoxicity mediated by soluble products of activated T cell lines. J Neuroimmunol 35:261-271
16. D'Souza SD, Bonetti B, Balasingam V et al (1996) Multiple sclerosis: Fas signaling in oligodendrocyte cell death. J Exp Med 184:2361-2370
17. Matysiak M, Jurewicz A, Jaskolski D, Selmaj K (2002) TRAIL induces death of human oligodendrocytes isolated from adult brain. Brain 125:2469-2480
18. Jurewicz A, Biddison WE, Antel JP (1998) MHC-class I-restricted lysis of human oligodendrocytes by myelin basic protein peptide-specific CD8 T lymphocytes. J Immunol 160:3056-3059
19. Merrill JE, Scolding NJ (1999) Mechanisms of damage to myelin and oligodendrocytes and their relevance to disease. Neuropathol Appl Neurobiol 25:435-458
20. Lassmann H, Brück W, Lucchinetti C, Rodriguez M (1997) Remyelination in multiple sclerosis. Mult Scler 3:133-136
21. Prineas JW, Connell F (1979) Remyelination in multiple sclerosis. Ann Neurol 5:22-31
22. Brück W, Schmied M, Suchanek G et al (1994) Oligodendrocytes in the early course of multiple sclerosis. Ann Neurol 35:65-73
23. Prineas JW, Barnard RO, Kwon EE et al (1993) Multiple sclerosis: remyelination of nascent lesions. Ann Neurol 33:137-151
24. Raine CS, Scheinberg L, Waltz JM (1981) Multiple sclerosis. Oligodendrocyte survival and proliferation in an active established lesion. Lab Invest 45:534-546
25. Lucchinetti CF, Brück W, Rodriguez M, Lassmann H (1996) Distinct patterns of multiple sclerosis pathology indicates heterogeneity in pathogenesis. Brain Pathol 6:259-274
26. Kornek B, Lassmann H (1999) Axonal pathology in multiple sclerosis. A historical note. Brain Pathol 9:651-656
27. Mews I, Bergmann M, Bunkowski S et al (1998) Oligodendrocyte and axon pathology in clinically silent multiple sclerosis lesions. Mult Scler 4:5-62
28. Lovas G, Szilágyi N, Komoly S et al (2000) Axonal changes in chronic demyelinated cervical spinal cord plaques. Brain 123:308-317
29. Kuhlmann T, Lingfeld G, Bitsch A et al (2002) Acute axonal damage in multiple sclerosis is most extensive in early disease stages and decreases over time. Brain 125:2202-2212
30. Allen IV, McKeown SR (1979) A histological, histochemical and biochemical study of the macroscopically normal white matter in multiple sclerosis. J Neurol Sci 41:81-91
31. Tartaglia MC, Narayanan S, De Stefano N et al (2002) Choline is increased in prelesional normal appearing white matter in multiple sclerosis. J Neurol 249:1382-1390
32. Allen IV, McQuaid S, Mirakhur M, Nevin G (2001) Pathological abnormalities in the normal-appearing white matter in multiple sclerosis. Neurol Sci 22:141-144

33. Gobin SJ, Montagne L, van Zutphen M et al (2001) Upregulation of transcription factors controlling MHC expression in multiple sclerosis lesions. Glia 36:68-77
34. Gveric D, Hanemaaijer R, Newcombe J et al (2001) Plasminogen activators in multiple sclerosis lesions. Implications for the inflammatory response and axonal damage. Brain 124:1978-1988
35. Lindberg RLP, De Groot CJA, Montagne L et al (2001) The expression profile of matrix metalloproteinases (MMPs) and their inhibitors (TIMPs) in lesions and normal appearing white matter of multiple sclerosis. Brain 124:1743-1753
36. Plumb J, McQuaid S, Mirakhur M, Kirk J (2002) Abnormal endothelial tight junctions in active lesions and normal-appearing white matter in multiple sclerosis. Brain Pathol 12:154-169
37. Kirk J, Plumb J, Mirakhur M, McQuaid S (2003) Tight junctional abnormality in multiple sclerosis white matter affects all calibres of vessel and is associated with blood-brain barrier leakage and active demyelination. J Pathol 201:319-327
38. Trapp BD, Peterson J, Ransohoff RM et al (1998) Axonal transection in the lesions of multiple sclerosis. New Engl J Med 338:278-285
39. Bitsch A, Schuchardt J, Bunkowski S et al (2000) Acute axonal injury in multiple sclerosis. Correlation with demyelination and inflammation. Brain 123:1174-1183
40. Waller A (1850) Experiments on the section of the glossopharyngeal and hypoglossal nerves of the frog, and observations of the alterations produced thereby in the structure of their primitive fibers. Phil Trans R Soc Lond (Biol) 140:423-429
41. Brück W (1997) The role of macrophages in Wallerian degeneration. Brain Pathol 7:741-752
42. Bjartmar C, Kinkel PR, Kidd G et al (2001) Axonal loss in normal-appearing white matter in a patient with acute MS. Neurology 57:1248-1252
43. Evangelou N, Esiri MM, Smith S et al (2000) Quantitative pathological evidence for axonal loss in normal appearing white matter in multiple sclerosis. Ann Neurol 47:391-395
44. Evangelou N, Konz D, Esiri MM et al (2000) Regional axonal loss in the corpus callosum correlates with cerebral white matter lesion volume and distribution in multiple sclerosis. Brain 123:845-1849
45. Ganter P, Prince C, Esiri MM (1999) Spinal cord axonal loss in multiple sclerosis: a post-mortem study. Neuropathol Appl Neurobiol 25:459-467
46. Giordana MT, Richiardi P, Trevisan E, Boghi A, Palmucci L (2002) Abnormal ubiquitination of axons in normally myelinated white matter in multiple sclerosis brain. Neuropathol Appl Neurobiol 28:35-41
47. Fu L, Matthews PM, De Stefano N et al (1998) Imaging axonal damage of normal appearing white matter in multiple sclerosis. Brain 121:103-113
48. Casanova B, Martinez-Bisbal MC, Valero C et al (2003) Evidence of Wallerian degeneration in normal appearing white matter in the early stages of relapsing-remitting multiple sclerosis. A 1HMRS study. J Neurol 250:22-28
49. Itoyama Y, Sternberger NH, Webster HD (1980) Immunocytochemical observations on the distribution of myelin associated glycoprotein and myelin basic protein in multiple sclerosis lesions. Ann Neurol 7:167-177
50. Wilczak N, De Keyser J (1997) Insulin-like growth factor-I receptors in normal appearing white matter and chronic plaques in multiple sclerosis. Brain Res 772:243-246

Chapter 2

Measurement of Blood-Brain Barrier Permeability in Multiple Sclerosis

D. Soon, D. Miller

Introduction

The concept of a barrier between the blood and the brain first arose in the late nineteenth century, when German bacteriologist Paul Ehrlich, discovered that aniline dyes injected intravenously into small animals stained all their organs except for the brain. The concept was developed further by his student, Goldman, who in 1905 demonstrated that tryptan blue injected intrathecally, but not intravenously, resulted in the staining of brain tissue. In the intervening century, histopathological and radiological investigations have helped shape our understanding of the blood-brain barrier (BBB) in health and in disease. In particular, the involvement of the BBB in neuroinflammation and how its disruption contributes to pathology is the subject of considerable study. This chapter will describe some of the principles and methods employed in the ongoing research making use of gadolinium (Gd)-enhanced magnetic resonance imaging (MRI) to investigate BBB disruption in multiple sclerosis (MS).

Structure and Function of the BBB in Health

The BBB serves a homoeostatic, protective function, maintaining a stable environment for optimum neuronal activity. It provides an anatomical and biochemical barrier to the influx of neurotransmitters and potential toxins from the bloodstream. In health, it helps maintain the brain as an immunologically privileged site [1]. It regulates the traffic of substances between the brain and the bloodstream through receptor-mediated transport, pinocytosis, and passive diffusion, allowing the influx of energy substrates and essential amino acids, and the efflux of metabolites.

The BBB exists in more than 99% of the capillaries of the brain [2], covering a considerable surface area of 180 cm^2/g brain tissue. In certain areas, it is replaced by a blood-CSF barrier, which, although more permeable than the BBB, still prevents the entry of many bloodborne compounds into the brain. This occurs in areas which serve a neurosecretory function, such as the posterior pituitary, and in areas which perform a chemoreceptive function, such as the circumventricular organs.

Histologically, the BBB consists of an epithelial-like endothelial layer, a basement membrane, attendant perivascular macrophages, pericytes, and astrocytes. The endothelial cells are characterized by intercellular junctions known as tight junctions, which consist structurally of multiple protein bands binding the membranes of adjacent cells. These tight junctions form the anatomical basis for the BBB, achieving a transendothelial electrical resistance of 1500 Ω/cm^2 [3] compared with the transendothelial resistance in systemic capillaries of 5-10 Ω/cm^2. The lack of fenestrations between neighbouring endothelial cells and the relative sparseness of pinocytic vesicles (that is, membrane-bound bodies by which substances can be transported through the cell) also contribute to the low transcellular permeability of the BBB. Ensheathing up to 90% of the abluminal surface of the endothelium are the foot processes of the astrocytes. Studies indicate that astrocytes induce the BBB phenotype in brain capillaries, probably through secreted factors [4, 5]. Astrocytes are also thought to confer a degree of protection over the endothelial layer against hypoxic and hypoglycaemic injury [6].

BBB Disruption

Table 1 details some of a growing number of conditions in which there is evidence of BBB disruption.

BBB disruption occurs in the two most common intracranial malignancies, that is, high-grade gliomas and metastatic adenocarcinoma. The disruption of the BBB leads to the vasogenic oedema which contributes to the morbidity and mortality associated with these tumours. Microvessels in metastatic adenocarcinomas are phenotypically similar to vessels in the tissue from which the tumours are derived. They therefore do not form tight junctions [13]. The mechanism for the breakdown of the BBB in gliomas is less certain. One possibility is that the loss of differentiation in glial cells causes a disruption of the secretion of factors necessary to maintain the BBB. An alternative explanation is that gliomas display accelerated angiogenesis associated with high levels of VEGF (vascular endothelial growth factor); this molecule has also been shown to influence permeability of microvessels [7].

Disruption of the BBB also appears to occur in sepsis, as evidenced by the detection of various bloodborne markers in the CSF [14, 15]. Microscopically,

Table 1. Conditions in which BBB disruption occurs

Multiple sclerosis
Tumours [7]
Trauma [8]
Infection [9]
Ischaemic injury [10]
Alzheimer's disease [11]
Epileptic seizures
Systemic illness – diabetes mellitus [12]

this is associated with swelling of astrocytic end feet, neuronal degeneration, and microvessel oedema [16]. The presence of BBB disruption in ischaemia is well documented, and vasogenic oedema frequently follows ischaemia-reperfusion events.

The involvement of the BBB in MS and the investigation of this using dynamic contrast imaging form the focus of this chapter.

Evidence of BBB Disruption in MS Lesions

Tryptan blue dye injected supravitally has provided evidence of detectable BBB disruption, mainly in acute lesions, but also to a lesser degree in chronic lesions [17]. Histological studies in the 1980s demonstrated perivenular fibrinous exudates and lymphocytic infiltration in acute and to a lesser extent chronic lesions, providing histological evidence of both BBB leakage and inflammation in MS lesions [18].

Gadolinium is a strongly paramagnetic element. It enhances the relaxation of surrounding protons, and therefore is associated with a high signal on T_1-weighted MRI. In its chelated forms, such as gadopentate dimeglumine (Gd-DTPA) [19], it has been used widely in MRI as an extracellular tracer.

In a combined MRI-pathology study of experimental allergic encephalitis (EAE) – an animal model for MS – Gd enhancement in lesions was correlated with histopathological evidence for BBB breakdown using the marker horseradish peroxidase [20]. The presence of Gd enhancement was also correlated with active inflammation, i.e. perivascular lymphocyte infiltrates.

Correlative histopathological-MRI studies in subjects with MS have demonstrated that Gd-enhancing lesions consistently demonstrate features of inflammation, e.g. perivascular lymphocytes and macrophage infiltrates [21, 22]. In vivo studies reveal that Gd enhancement is a regular finding in new lesions. The duration of enhancement in new lesions as well as the pattern of enhancement have been shown to be heterogeneous, with ring enhancement, patchy, and nodular enhancement all being observed [23], and with serial scans demonstrating enhancement over a range of durations, most often between 2 and 8 weeks [24-26]. Chronic lesions may also visibly enhance on Gd administration [27], although this is a much less common event. By increasing the dosage of Gd and modifying the sequences used, it is possible to detect significantly more MS lesions with BBB breakdown [28, 29].

A recent study examined more subtle BBB leakage quantitatively. The mean signal intensity of lesions was measured at various times points on T_1-weighted spin echo images before and after the administration of triple-dose Gd. Significant post-contrast signal increase was demonstrated in focal, non-visibly enhancing lesions when compared against anatomically analogous contralateral normal-appearing white matter (NAWM). The results of the study are shown in Table 2. The significant difference in enhancement seen in NAWM and in

Table 2. Median percentage change in signal intensity in all MS lesions compared with anatomically analogous contralateral NAWM. Figures in parentheses indicate interquartile range. (From [30], with permission)

Time after Gd administration	NAWM	All MS lesions	*p* value
5 min	1.9 (0.3 to 3.6)	3.2 (0.9 to 5.5)	$p<0.0005$
20 min	1.2 (–0.8 to +0.31)	2.5 (–0.2 to +5.1)	$p<0.0005$
40 min	0.7 (–1.3 to +2.7)	1.8 (–1.0 to +4.6)	$p<0.0005$

MS lesions suggests incomplete BBB repair in chronic lesions, leading to subtle leakage [30].

BBB Disruption in the NAWM

Some recent histological studies suggest that there may be subtle BBB disruption in the NAWM secondary to the degradation of tight junctions [31, 32]. While no radiological study to date has been able to demonstrate BBB leakage in the NAWM of MS patients, a non-significant trend toward enhancement was seen in the NAWM of MS patients when compared with healthy controls after the administration of triple-dose Gd [30].

Table 3 illustrates the median proportional change in signal intensity in the NAWM of healthy controls and of MS patients. As can be seen, the only significant change is seen in the healthy controls in the first 5 min after administration of Gd. This is thought to be attributable to the presence of intravascular Gd, and the short-lived nature of this initial enhancement is consistent with the intravascular half-life of Gd [33]. There is also a non-significant, persistent trend toward signal intensity increase seen in the NAWM of MS patients, suggesting a very subtle leakage.

Quantitative MRI studies using a number of measures have indicated the presence of abnormality within NAWM [34-38]. T_1 has been shown to be prolonged in NAWM compared with healthy controls [39], suggesting the presence of excess water. One mechanism for this would be BBB disruption, although other intrinsic pathological changes in NAWM might also be associated with an increase in water content.

Table 3. Median percentage change in signal intensity in the NAWM of healthy controls and MS patients. Figures in parentheses indicate interquartile range. (From [30], with permission)

Time after Gd administration	Healthy controls	MS patients
5 min	1.8* (0.5 to 3.2)	1.5 (–0.1 to +2.8)
20 min	0.1 (–1.1 to +1.8)	1.0 (–0.9 to +2.5)
40 min	–1.3 (–1.5 to +1.2)	0.4 (–1.6 to +2.2)

*$p<0.0005$

A meta-analysis of short-term serial Gd-enhanced studies on relapsing-remitting MS and secondary progressive MS has shown that the number of new Gd-enhancing lesions is a poor predictor of clinical outcome [40]. In primary progressive MS, clinical disability is frequently marked despite the relative paucity of new lesions [41]. A question therefore arises whether there might exist a more subtle BBB leakage in both NAWM and chronically visibly non-enhancing lesions, which may account for low-grade inflammation and clinical progression which is not explained by the presence of actively inflamed (Gd-enhancing) lesions.

Principles of BBB Permeability Calculation

The change in T_1 relaxation time following Gd administration is related to Gd concentration $C_t(t)$ by the following equation:

$$C_t(t) = \frac{\frac{1}{T_1} - \frac{1}{T_{10}}}{r_1},$$

where T_1 is the T_1 relaxation time at the time *t* after Gd administration, T_{10} the T_1 relaxation time before Gd administration, or native T_1. r_1 is the relaxivity of Gd, which for Gd-DTPA is estimated as 4.5 $s^{-1}mM^{-1}$ [42, 43].

The plasma concentration of Gd C_p can be estimated using the four-compartment model [43]. This assumes a distribution of Gd between plasma, the extracellular space, the lesion leakage space, and the kidneys (Fig. 1). Using this mod-

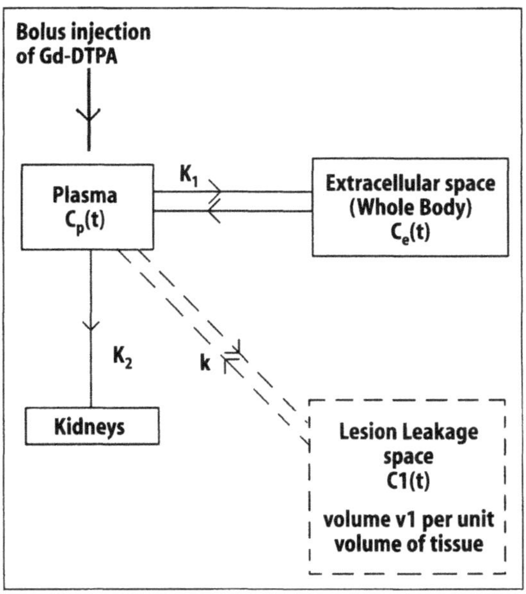

Fig. 1. The four-compartment model of Gd distribution. From[42]

el, the concentration of Gd in plasma follows a biexponential curve, in which Gd is lost into the kidneys and into the extravascular, extracellular space (EES) of the body outside the brain.

$$Cp(t) = D\,\{a_1 \exp(-m_1 t) + a2 \exp(-m2t)\},$$

where D is the dose of Gd, a_1 and a_2 are the amplitudes, and m_1 and m_2 are the rate constants of the two components (a fast component representing the equilibration of Gd with the EES and a slow component representing the loss of Gd into the kidneys).

Having modelled the concentration of Gd in plasma, and in assuming that flow is proportional to the surface area of the leaking membrane and the concentration difference across the membrane, it is possible to estimate the permeability surface area product PS and the leakage space $v_1 V_1$, that is, the space into which Gd leaks, using the following equation:

$$v_1 V_1 \frac{dC_t}{dt} = PS(C_p - C_t),$$

where V_1 is the volume of tissue looked at and v_1 the proportion of the tissue making up the leakage space. Or, in other words:

$$v_1 \frac{dC_t}{dt} = k(C_p - C_t),$$

where $k=PS/V_t$, the permeability surface area product per unit volume of tissue, otherwise known as the transfer coefficient. Using this model, permeability has been measured in MS lesions [42] and after ischaemia and reperfusion in rat brain [44] and in gliomas [45].

Quantification of Scanner Variability

Positron emission tomography (PET) studies using ^{68}Ga-EDTA obtained permeability PS values of $3.0 \pm 0.8 \cdot 10^{-4}$ min^{-1} [46, 47]. Based on these values, and assuming a T_1 relaxation time of 600 ms, an extravascular extracellular space of $v_1=0.15$ and a relaxivity of Gd to be 4.5 s^{-1} mM^{-1}, leakage through intact capillaries in healthy controls should translate to a reduction in T_1 of 23 ms (4%) over 1 h following the injection of a triple dose of Gd (personal communication, P. Tofts 2003). It was therefore important to quantify and characterize scanner variability during serial scanning experiments over a period of 1 h (a time span comparable to the duration of our planned experiments with triple-dose Gd) to see whether the detection of such small changes was feasible on the current scanner. We considered three possible candidate scan sequences which would conceivably detect subtle changes in T_1 relaxation time and hence small changes in Gd concentration, which we would then employ to measure permeability in volunteer patients and controls. The selection of the sequence was based on a number of criteria including sensitivity, stability, reproducibility, and acquisition time.

MRI Protocol

All imaging was carried out using a 1.5-T superconducting system with standard quadrature headcoil (Signa, GE Medical Systems, Milwaukee, Wis.). A single healthy subject was scanned on eight separate occasions, each session involving three cycles of four sequences, to determine which sequence would be associated with the least scanner variability and the best reproducibility. They are shown in Table 4.

The T_1 gradient echo and proton density (PD) gradient echo sequences are utilized in determining T_1 relaxation times and in the construction of a T_1 map using a technique developed in-house [48], which employs a knowledge of the RF pulse profile and a map of the coil transmission B_1 distribution, where B_1 is the magnetic field as applied by the RF pulse, to avoid errors introduced by slice profile or coil non-uniformity.

Analysis

Following acquisition, all images were transferred to a Sun Workstation (Sun Microsystems, Mountain View, Calif., USA) on which all further analysis was performed. The images were segmented into white and grey matter constituents using SPM 99 (Statistical Parametric Mapping; Wellcome Department of Cognitive Neurology, Institute of Neurology, Queen Square, London) [49], and the mean intensities of the whole brain parenchyma as well as grey and white matter segments were determined by the application of histograms to the constituents.

Table 4. Parameters for sequences used to characterize scan variability

Sequence	T_1-weighted spin echo	3D fast spoiled gradient echo	T_1 gradient echo sequence	Proton-density gradient echo sequence
Repetition time	600 ms	13.3 ms	1500 ms	50 ms
Echo time	17 ms	4.2 ms	11 ms	11 ms
Inversion time	–	450 ms	–	–
Number of slices	46	124	25	25
Slice thickness	3 mm	1.5 mm	5 mm	5 mm
Flip angle	90	20	45	45
Matrix	256×256	256×256	256×256	256×256
Field of view	240×240	300×225	256×128	256×128
Duration	6 min	8 min	8 min	8 min

Results

The study is ongoing and we now report our findings to date. A consistent – and as yet unexplained – finding has been a drift in quantitative T_1 signal intensity and relaxation time measurements over the hour of repeated scanning of a healthy control without using contrast. With regard to the T_1-weighted sequences, the time-averaged relative drift for the T_1 gradient echo, T_1-weighted spin echo and 3D spoiled gradient recall (SPGR) sequences are shown in Table 5. The T_1-weighted gradient echo sequence exhibits a significantly lower drift than the other two sequences ($p=0.05$ and 0.01 for T_1-weighted spin echo and 3D SPGR respectively using a paired t-test). Figure 2 illustrates the proportional drift associated with each of the candidate sequences. As can be seen, the T_1 gradient echo sequence is associated with a much smaller drift than the other two sequences over the course of 1 h.

T_1 gradient echo sequence is used together with a PD-weighted gradient echo sequence to calculate T_1 relaxation [48]. This method relates the ratio ($R(T_1)$) of

Table 5. Relative drift in whole brain mean intensities in T1-weighted MRI sequences over three repeated cycles

	T1-weighted GE drift (%)	T1-weighted SE drift (%)	3D SPGR drift (%)
1st cycle	0	0	0
2nd cycle (35 min)	–0.65108	–1.45029	–2.195106
3rd cycle (70 min)	–1.17841	–2.34762	–2.857724

SPGR, spoiled gradient recall

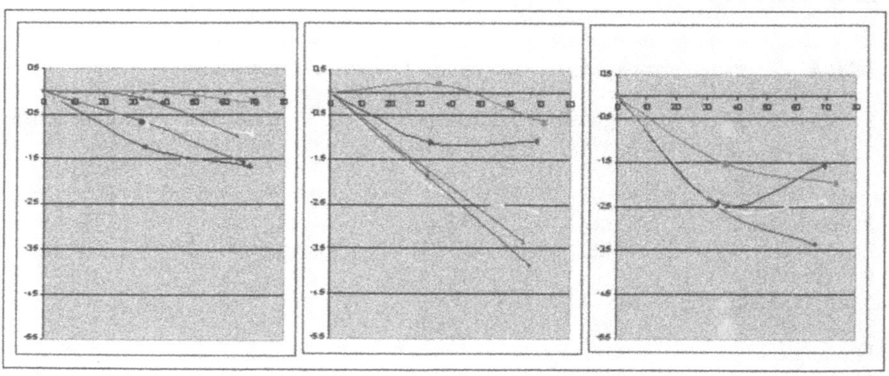

Fig. 2. Relative drift over time in T_1-weighted sequences. From *left* to *right:* T_1 gradient echo, T_1-weighted spin echo, 3D SPGR

T_1-weighted signal intensity (S_{T1W}) and PD-weighted signal intensity (S_{PDW}) to T_1 relaxation time, using a lookup table which takes into account the radiofrequency pulse non-uniformity and inconsistencies in the magnetic field.

$$R(T_1) = \frac{S_{T1W}}{S_{PDW}},$$

T_1 relaxation time is inversely related to $R(T_1)$, that is T_1 relaxation time is inversely related to T_1-weighted signal intensity and directly related to PD-weighted signal intensity.

Studies on the drift of PD-weighted signal intensity revealed an average significant drift in signal intensity of –2.5% at 35 min and –3.5% at 70 min (Fig. 3). Because this drift is larger in magnitude than the drift in T_1-weighted signal intensity, the calculated T_1 relaxation time accordingly follows a downward trend owing to the larger influence of the PD-weighted image.

Figure 4 shows the change in calculated T_1 relaxation time on a normal subject following repeated measurements using repeated PD cycles. At 60 min, the predicted drift is –35.7 ms with a 95% confidence upper limit of –22.3 ms and a lower limit of –49.1 ms (thus an error of ±15 ms).

Assuming that PD does not vary in the human brain, and exploring the possibility of calculating T_1 based on the initial PD-weighted image, the curves shown in Fig. 5 are obtained. Because the calculated T_1 relaxation curve is no longer affected by the downward drift of serial PD-weighted images, the resultant drift of T_1 time reflects the drift of T_1-weighted gradient echo, and hence displays an upward trend. In addition, because the variation in PD-weighted signal intensity is removed, there is much less variation in the resultant T_1 relaxation time curve, with narrower confidence margins. In this case, the predicted drift at 60 min is 30.8 ms with an upper limit of normal 39.1 ms and a lower limit of normal being 22.1 ms (an error of ±10ms).

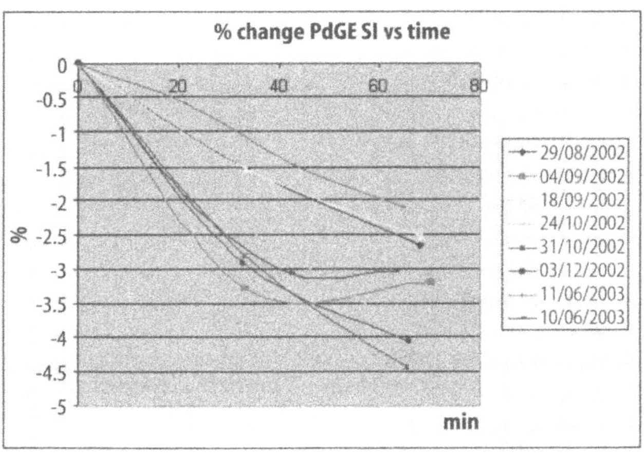

Fig. 3. Relative drift in signal intensity in proton density-weighted gradient echo sequence against time in minutes

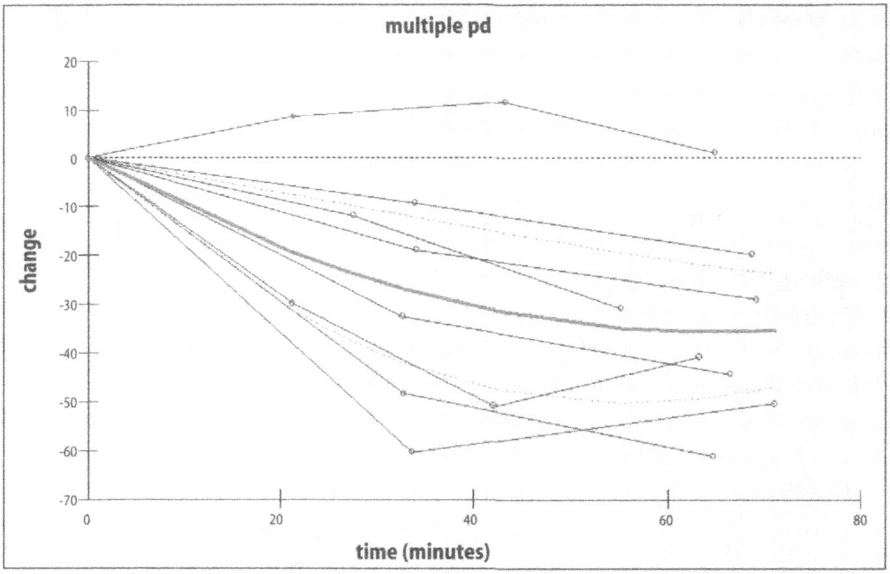

Fig. 4. Drift (milliseconds) in calculated T_1 relaxation time for whole brain vs scanning time (minutes), using repeated proton density measurements to ascertain the T_1 relaxation time at each time point. The average drift is represented in the *bold red line*, and the *dotted red lines* represent the 95% confidence intervals. At 60 min, the predicted drift is –35.7 ms, with a 95% confidence upper limit of –22.3 ms and a lower limit of –49.1 ms (thus an error of ±15 ms)

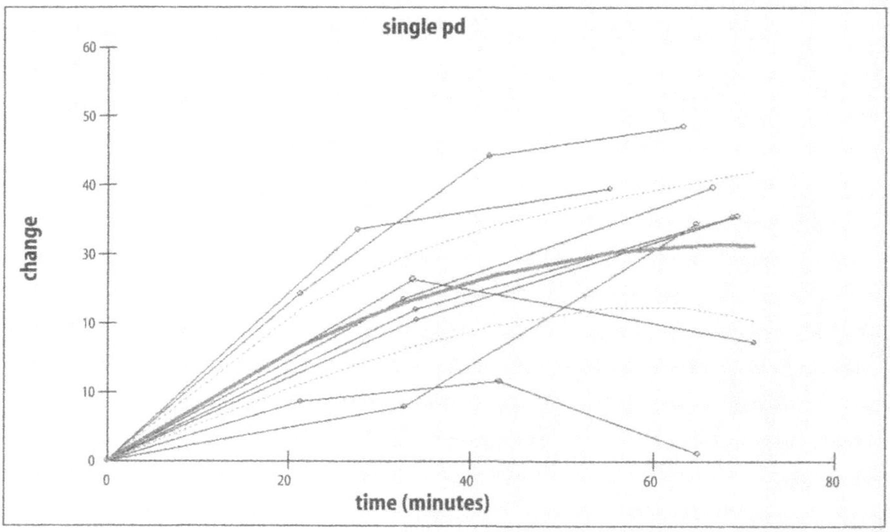

Fig. 5. Drift in calculated T_1 relaxation time (milliseconds) vs scanning time (minutes) using a single proton-density-weighted sequence at the beginning of the repeated cycles to calculate T_1 relaxation time. The *bold red line* represents the average drift over time, and the *dotted red lines* represent the 95% confidence intervals

Work is still going on to detect sources of the drift and devise strategies to minimize it. In order to detect the leakage of Gd in a healthy control, the scanner should be sensitive enough to detect changes in T_1 relaxation time of the order of 20 ms in 1 h. While drift in calculated T_1 relaxation time reaches about twice this value, the usage of a single PD-weighted image to calculate T_1 has resulted in lower variation of the drift gradient, enabling a more certain characterization of drift, which can then be used to correct measured data (within ±10 ms). Moreover the BBB permeability in chronic, non-enhancing lesions is probably larger than in NAWM and has already been shown to result in changes of a magnitude detectable at current levels of scanner sensitivity [30]. The use of triple-dose Gd can also be used in looking at permeability changes in chronic lesions to determine whether certain therapeutic measures influence BBB permeability. This is being undertaken as a sub-study in the current placebo-controlled trial of the anti-adhesion molecule antibody natalizumab (a VLA4 antagonist).

We are currently acquiring data for a cross-sectional study of various MS subgroups. In this study, we measure and plot the change in T_1 relaxation time before and after the administration of triple-dose Gd. Preliminary studies on the four secondary progressive and two relapsing remitting patients scanned thus far indicate an observable change in the T_1 relaxation time in chronic non-visibly-enhancing lesions. This change is of the order of 100 ms and is much larger than the drift observed in our studies of scanner variability. The change is also significantly different from anatomically analogous regions of interest described in the contralateral NAWM (p=0.015). Relative change in signal intensity of T_1-weighted gradient echo shows a change of 2%-5% after Gd administration, which is broadly in agreement with the recent study looking at quantitative enhancement with T_1-weighted spin echo in lesions [30].

We thus find ourselves in a position where we can map and characterize BBB permeability in chronic, non-enhancing lesions. The next step would be to focus on the NAWM BBB disruption suggested at by histological and radiological studies. A high level of scanner stability and sequence sensitivity and reproducibility will be required if we are to measure and characterize the BBB permeability of NAWM satisfactorily within various MS subtypes.

Acknowledgements. We would like to thank the following people for their invaluable help and advice: Professor Paul Tofts, Dr Daniel Altmann, Dr Daniel Tozer, Dr Claudia Wheeler- Kingshott, Dr Nicholas Silver. The MS NMR Unit is supported by the MS Society of Great Britain and Northern Ireland. DS is supported by Biogen.

References

1. Pachter JS, de Vries HE, Fabry Z (2003) The blood-brain barrier and its role in immune privilege in the central nervous system. J Neuropathol Exp Neurol 62:593-604
2. de Vries HE, Kuiper J, de Boer AG et al (1997) The blood-brain barrier in neuroinflammatory diseases. Pharmacol Rev 49:143-155

3. Butt AM, Jones HC, Abbott NJ (1990) Electrical resistance across the blood-brain barrier in anaesthetized rats: a developmental study. J Physiol 429:47-62
4. Janzer RC, Raff MC (1987) Astrocytes induce blood-brain barrier properties in endothelial cells. Nature 325:253-257
5. Sobue K, Yamamoto N, Yoneda K et al (1999) Induction of blood-brain barrier properties in immortalized bovine brain endothelial cells by astrocytic factors. Neurosci Res 35:155-164
6. Abbruscato TJ, Davis TP (1999) Protein expression of brain endothelial cell E-cadherin after hypoxia/aglycemia: influence of astrocyte contact. Brain Res 842:277-286
7. Davies DC (2002) Blood-brain barrier breakdown in septic encephalopathy and brain tumours. J Anat 200:639-646
8. Povlishock JT, Becker DP, Sullivan HG et al (1978) Vascular permeability alterations to horseradish peroxidase in experimental brain injury. Brain Res 153:223-239
9. Clawson CC, Hartmann JF, Vernier RL (1966) Electron microscopy of the effect of gram-negative endotoxin on the blood-brain barrier. J Comp Neurol 127:183-198
10. Kuroiwa T, Shibutani M, Okeda R (1988) Blood-brain barrier disruption and exacerbation of ischemic brain edema after restoration of blood flow in experimental focal cerebral ischemia. Acta Neuropathol (Berl) 76:62-70
11. Berzin TM, Zipser BD, Rafii MS et al (2000) Agrin and microvascular damage in Alzheimer's disease. Neurobiol Aging 21:349-355
12. Mooradian AD (1997) Central nervous system complications of diabetes mellitus – a perspective from the blood-brain barrier. Brain Res Brain Res Rev 23:210-218
13. Long DM (1979) Capillary ultrastructure in human metastatic brain tumors. J Neurosurg 51:53-58
14. Deng X, Wang X, Andersson R (1995) Endothelial barrier resistance in multiple organs after septic and nonseptic challenges in the rat. J Appl Physiol 78:2052-2061
15. Jeppsson B, Freund HR, Gimmon Z et al (1981) Blood-brain barrier derangement in sepsis: cause of septic encephalopathy? Am J Surg 141:136-142
16. Papadopoulos MC, Lamb FJ, Moss RF et al (1999) Faecal peritonitis causes oedema and neuronal injury in pig cerebral cortex. Clin Sci (Lond) 96:461-466
17. Broman T (1964) Blood-brain barrier damage in multiple sclerosis supravital test-observations. Acta Neurol Scand 40:Suppl 4
18. Adams CW, Poston RN, Buk SJ et al (1985) Inflammatory vasculitis in multiple sclerosis. J Neurol Sci 69:269-283
19. Mitchell DG (1997) MR imaging contrast agents – what's in a name? J Magn Reson Imaging 7:1-4
20. Hawkins CP, Munro PM, Mackenzie F et al (1990) Duration and selectivity of blood-brain barrier breakdown in chronic relapsing experimental allergic encephalomyelitis studied by gadolinium-DTPA and protein markers. Brain 113:365-378
21. Katz D, Taubenberger JK, Cannella B et al (1993) Correlation between magnetic resonance imaging findings and lesion development in chronic, active multiple sclerosis. Ann Neurol 34:661-669
22. Bruck W, Bitsch A, Kolenda H et al (1997) Inflammatory central nervous system demyelination: correlation of magnetic resonance imaging findings with lesion pathology. Ann Neurol 42:783-793
23. Kermode AG, Tofts PS, Thompson AJ et al (1990) Heterogeneity of blood-brain barrier changes in multiple sclerosis: an MRI study with gadolinium-DTPA enhancement. Neurology 40:229-235
24. Miller DH, Rudge P, Johnson G et al (1988) Serial gadolinium enhanced magnetic resonance imaging in multiple sclerosis. Brain 111:927-939
25. Tortorella C, Codella M, Rocca MA et al (1999) Disease activity in multiple sclerosis studied by weekly triple-dose magnetic resonance imaging. J Neurol 246:689-692

26. Cotton F, Weiner HL, Jolesz FA et al (2003) MRI contrast uptake in new lesions in relapsing-remitting MS followed at weekly intervals. Neurology 60:640-646
27. Barnes D, Munro PM, Youl BD et al (1991) The longstanding MS lesion. A quantitative MRI and electron microscopic study. Brain 114:1271-1280
28. Filippi M, Yousry T, Campi A et al (1996) Comparison of triple dose versus standard dose gadolinium-DTPA for detection of MRI enhancing lesions in patients with MS. Neurology 46:379-384
29. Silver NC, Good CD, Barker GJ et al (1997) Sensitivity of contrast enhanced MRI in multiple sclerosis. Effects of gadolinium dose, magnetization transfer contrast and delayed imaging. Brain 120:1149-1161
30. Silver NC, Tofts PS, Symms MR et al (2001) Quantitative contrast-enhanced magnetic resonance imaging to evaluate blood-brain barrier integrity in multiple sclerosis: a preliminary study. Mult Scler 7:75-82
31. Plumb J, McQuaid S, Mirakhur M et al (2002) Abnormal endothelial tight junctions in active lesions and normal-appearing white matter in multiple sclerosis. Brain Pathol 12:154-169
32. Kirk J, Plumb J, Mirakhur M et al (2003) Tight junctional abnormality in multiple sclerosis white matter affects all calibres of vessel and is associated with blood-brain barrier leakage and active demyelination. J Pathol 201:319-327
33. Niendorf (1994) Safety and risk of gadolinium- DTPA: extended clinical experience after more than 5,000,000 appliations. Magnevist. Blackwell Scientific Publications, pp 5-14
34. Filippi M, Campi A, Dousset V et al (1995) A magnetization transfer imaging study of normal-appearing white matter in multiple sclerosis. Neurology 45:478-482
35. Losseff NA, Wang L, Lai HM et al (1996) Progressive cerebral atrophy in multiple sclerosis. A serial MRI study. Brain 119:2009-2019
36. Kidd D, Barker GJ, Tofts PS et al (1997) The transverse magnetisation decay characteristics of longstanding lesions and normal-appearing white matter in multiple sclerosis. J Neurol 244:125-130
37. Werring DJ, Brassat D, Droogan AG et al (2000) The pathogenesis of lesions and normal-appearing white matter changes in multiple sclerosis: a serial diffusion MRI study. Brain 123:1667-1676
38. Chard DT, Griffin CM, McLean MA et al (2002) Brain metabolite changes in cortical grey and normal-appearing white matter in clinically early relapsing-remitting multiple sclerosis. Brain 125:2342-2352
39. Griffin CM, Dehmeshki J, Chard DT et al (2002) T1 histograms of normal-appearing brain tissue are abnormal in early relapsing-remitting multiple sclerosis. Mult Scler 8:211-216
40. Kappos L, Moeri D, Radue EW et al (1999) Predictive value of gadolinium-enhanced magnetic resonance imaging for relapse rate and changes in disability or impairment in multiple sclerosis: a meta-analysis. Gadolinium MRI Meta-analysis Group. Lancet 353:964-969
41. Thompson AJ, Kermode AG, Wicks D et al (1991) Major differences in the dynamics of primary and secondary progressive multiple sclerosis. Ann Neurol 29:53-62
42. Tofts PS, Kermode AG (1991) Measurement of the blood-brain barrier permeability and leakage space using dynamic MR imaging. 1. Fundamental concepts. Magn Reson Med 17:357-367
43. Tofts PS, Brix G, Buckley DL et al (1999) Estimating kinetic parameters from dynamic contrast-enhanced T(1)-weighted MRI of a diffusable tracer: standardized quantities and symbols. J Magn Reson Imaging 10:223-232
44. Harris NG, Gauden V, Fraser PA et al (2002) MRI measurement of blood-brain barrier permeability following spontaneous reperfusion in the starch microsphere model of ischemia. Magn Reson Imaging 20:221-230

45. Zhu XP, Li KL, Kamaly-Asl ID et al (2000) Quantification of endothelial permeability, leakage space, and blood volume in brain tumors using combined T1 and T2* contrast-enhanced dynamic MR imaging. J Magn Reson Imaging 11:575-585
46. Iannotti F, Fieschi C, Alfano B et al (1987) Simplified, noninvasive PET measurement of blood-brain barrier permeability. J Comput Assist Tomogr 11:390-397
47. Pozzilli C, Bernardi S, Mansi L et al (1988) Quantitative assessment of blood-brain barrier permeability in multiple sclerosis using 68-Ga-EDTA and positron emission tomography. J Neurol Neurosurg Psychiatry 51:1058-1062
48. Parker GJ, Barker GJ, Tofts PS (2001) Accurate multislice gradient echo T(1) measurement in the presence of non-ideal RF pulse shape and RF field nonuniformity. Magn Reson Med 45:838-845
49. Ashburner J, Friston K (1997) Multimodal image coregistration and partitioning – a unified framework. Neuroimage 6:209-217

Chapter 3

Measuring and Interpreting White Matter Volume Changes in Multiple Sclerosis

C. WEGNER, S. SMITH, P.M. MATTHEWS

Neuronal and Axonal Degeneration in Multiple Sclerosis

Neuronal and axonal degeneration have become recognized as major elements in the pathology of multiple sclerosis (MS). Interest has developed in monitoring these events in vivo with the recognition that they are closely coupled to development of disability [1]. A compelling question at present is the extent to which these phenomena are linked to the predominantly T-cell-mediated inflammatory changes in white matter ("plaques"), hitherto believed to be the pathological hallmark of MS.

The primary triggers for neuronal and axonal degeneration and loss in MS are not known, but there are several plausible links relating these events to primary white matter inflammation. Neuronal [2] and axonal [3] injury are found in regions of grey and white matter inflammation, respectively. Inflammation in MS could lead to a cascade of injury even if neurons and axons are not direct targets. Macrophages are activated, which could potentially lead to release of toxic cytokines. B cell activation with antibody production can lead to complement-mediated injury. There is widespread upregulation of nitric oxide synthase and release of nitric oxide, a potent inhibitor of mitochondrial respiration able to cause rapid functional impairment in axons and lead to neuronal death. However, neuronal [4] and axonal [5, 6] injury also are found in regions remote from inflammation. With more prolonged inflammation and damage, there may be epitope spreading, by which neurons may become direct targets. Alternative mechanisms of neurodegeneration are suggested by evidence that even with dramatic suppression of inflammation (at least in the later stages of clinical evolution), neuroaxonal injury may continue to progress [7].

Brain Atrophy in MS

A number of recent studies have directed attention to the possibility that measurement of brain atrophy can be used as an index of neuroaxonal injury in MS. Loss of myelin, axons, and neurons all would be expected to give rise to brain substance loss. It has long been recognized that late-stage MS is associated with substantial atrophy of the brain with marked ventriculomegaly. With the advent of high-quality magnetic resonance imaging (MRI) and digital signal processing methods, it has also become possible to measure even very small changes in brain volume occurring over relatively short periods in vivo (e.g. 6 months to 1 year or longer).

Serial MRI studies have concluded consistently that brain volume loss occurs at a faster rate in patients with MS than in age-matched, healthy controls.

Depending on the measuring method used, studies have reported reductions in brain volume by 0.6%-1% per year in MS patients [1, 8-10] (while brain volume in healthy controls is estimated to decrease by about 0.1%-0.3% per year) [11-13]. A recent study in normal subjects found a significant age-associated decrease in global (–0.3%/year) and regional brain volumes [14]. However, the changes in brain volume in MS occur from the earliest stages of the disease, even from the time of first presentation with a clinically isolated syndrome [15-17]. Atrophy appears to proceed inexorably through the course of the disease [18].

Interest has increased in brain atrophy measures for two primary reasons. Firstly, brain atrophy has been closely associated in several studies with the development of disability [1]. It therefore is considered to be a clinically relevant surrogate marker of disease progression. Secondly, as it can be assessed from serial T_1-weighted images, acquisition of the primary imaging data is possible on all scanners using already implemented protocols. In fact, atrophy can be reliably estimated from datasets acquired in the past, before this outcome measure had been planned to be used.

What Accounts for Brain Atrophy in MS?

The inflammatory lesions are most obvious in the white matter (although there remain a significant fraction that are found at the white matter/grey matter junction and in the grey matter itself). Probabilistic mapping of lesions across space over cohorts of patients with MS demonstrated very well how the lesions of MS tend to be clustered in a predominantly periventricular fashion involving the corpus callosum and descending cortical spinal tracts [19]. Enhancing lesions reflecting active inflammation were shown to be related to subsequent brain atrophy. This gives evidence for a cascade of potentially irreversible tissue damage that may follow inflammation and result in atrophy [20, 21]. Axonal transection occurs most obviously in regions of these prior inflammatory lesions. On T_1-weighted images, the "black holes" (which are correlated with loss of axonal substance [22]) are localized in previous regions of inflammation and with gliosis. These destructive changes must contribute to brain volume loss in the white matter, and cerebral atrophy was shown to be associated with an increased T_1-hypointense lesion load, but not with the total T_2 load [23, 24]. Changes in the normal-appearing white matter (NAWM) are also likely to contribute to overall atrophy. Evangelou and colleagues found a relationship between axonal density in the normal-appearing corpus callosum and cerebral hemisphere white matter lesion load, indicating that changes in the NAWM may be in part a consequence of Wallerian degeneration [5].

Axonal loss and demyelination will inevitably lead to tissue atrophy in MS. Myelin is estimated to constitute about 24% and axons about 46% of the volume of white matter [25]. Imaging evidence that atrophy in MS is associated with axonal loss comes from magnetic resonance spectroscopy studies showing that atrophy is associated with reduction of the neuronal marker *N*-acetylaspartate [26]. Loss of myelin must also contribute to brain volume loss in MS. It should be noted that even isolated demyelination should give rise to myelin loss, regardless of whether it is followed by remyelination, given the thinner myelin lamellae with the latter [27].

It may be useful to consider the potential relative contributions of these different tissue compartments to brain atrophy in MS quantitatively. Demyelination in focal white matter T_2-hyperintense lesions – to the extent typically seen in MS brains (e.g. volumes of 10-60 cm^3) – *alone* would be expected to give rise to only approximately 1% loss of total brain volume (100×[60 cm^3×0.24)/(1200 cm^3)]) (a 1200-cm^3 brain is assumed). If lesion volume grew by 10% per year, this would alone account for only a 0.1%/year rate of brain volume relatively. Although it is difficult to compare absolute measures of brain atrophy between different methods, this is only a relatively small proportion of that observed with methods that measure whole brain volume (e.g. SIENA) (Table 1; Fig. 1). This may be one factor that contributes to the

Table 1. Results from quantitative imaging studies of relative brain atrophy rate in multiple sclerosis and normal subjects. As methods and time periods of observation vary substantially, it is not possible to compare results obtained in different studies directly. However, there is general agreement that patients with multiple sclerosis show increased rates of relative brain volume loss over time

Approach	Method	Study	Measured atrophy	Normal subjects
Linear measures	Ventricle width	Simon et al. (1999) [20]	+4.5 to +5.5% ventricle width –0.64% brain width	
Semi-manual measures	Central cerebral volume	Losseff et al. (1996) [1]	–1.8 to –6.4 ml	
	Central cerebral volume	Molyneux et al. (2000) [21]	–0.97 to –1.3%	
	Central cerebral volume	Pfefferbaum et al. (1994) [12]	–	+0.3 ml ventricular volume
	Cavalieri	Liu et al. (1999) [9]	–12% to –21% estimate of volume loss	
Brain segmentation	BPF	Rudick et al. (1999) [8]	–0.55% BPF	
	BPF	Fisher et al. (2002) [18]	–0.55% BPF (years 1-2) –0.33% BPF (years 3-8)	
Brain registration	BBSI	Fox et al. (2000) [10]	–0.8% atrophy rate	–0.30%
	MIDAS	Brex et al. (2000) [17]	+ ≤0.8 cm^3 ventricular volume	
	MIDAS	Scahill et al. (2003) [14]	–	–0.32%
	SIENA	Stevenson et al. (2000) [43]	–0.57%	
	Central cerebral volume		–2.31%	

BPF, brain parenchymal fraction; *BICCR*, brain intracranial capacity ratio; *EBSI*, brain boundary shift integral; *MIDAS*, technique for measuring ventricular volume; *SIENA*, Structural Image Evaluation, using Normalization, of Atrophy

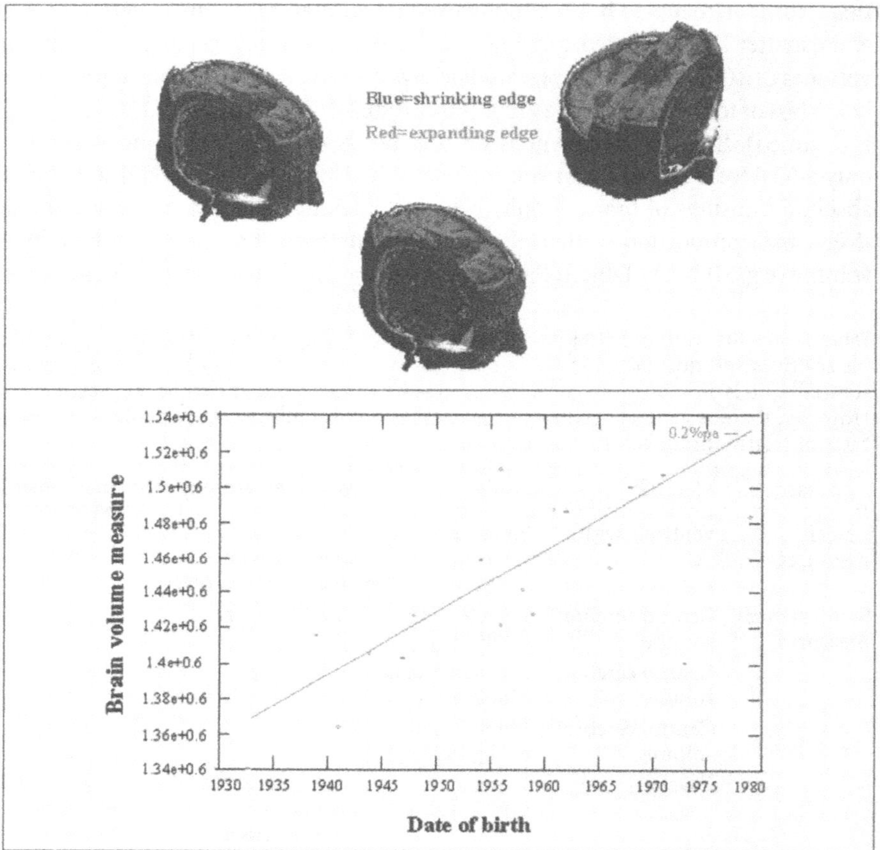

Fig. 1. In the *upper panel*, rendered brain volumes show changes in brain volume in a patient with MS over 2 years as measured with SIENA (www.fmrib.ox.ac.uk/fsl/). *Blue points* indicate relative atrophy and *red points* apparent "growth" (reflecting "noise" largely, e.g., from registration errors with relative movement of the brain between the two scans). The predominance of the blue edge points demonstrates that – overall – the brain is atrophying. The atrophy occurs particularly at the periphery of the cortex and around the ventricles. In the *lower panel*, the graph shows the age-associated decrease in global brain volume measured by SIENAX, a variant of SIENA (www.fmrib.ox.ac.uk/fsl), in healthy subjects. These data reveal a "physiological" atrophy rate of 0.2% per year in the healthy brain

poor relationship between T_2 lesion volume increases (reflecting demyelination, as well as oedema and gliosis) and the progression of atrophy.

Loss of axons in lesions could potentially give rise to as much as twice this contribution to annual rate of change. This is clearly an overestimate, however, as all axons are not lost from lesions in general. Even considering demyelination and axon loss in focal lesions together, therefore, we cannot account for the substantial rate of total loss of brain substance in patients with MS. We therefore can conclude that axon and myelin loss in lesions does not alone account for the atrophy observed. *A major proportion of the pathology reflected in the measurement of brain atrophy must occur in tissue that is normal-appearing by MRI.*

Direct histopathological observations in the corpus callosum in late-stage secondary progressive MS demonstrated loss of greater than 50% of axons even in the NAWM [6]. While there was also an expansion of the extra-axonal space, there was a net loss of volume of about 35%. The ratio of total volume loss to axonal loss in this region can be estimated as approximately 35%/50%=0.7. Over the course of the disease, therefore, an estimate of 100×(0.35×0.45%)=16% of the total volume loss is attributable to white matter volume loss. Over 40 years of this chronic disease, this would give a contribution of approximately 0.4%/year. This is larger than the typically expected contribution from axonal loss and demyelination *within* lesions. This relatively large rate of volume loss in NAWM can be rationalized both in terms of degeneration of axons (and secondary loss of myelin) from lesions and potential contributions from "microscopic" lesions scattered through the normal appearing tissue.

Atrophy of the grey matter could contribute a similar, additional amount to the total rate of volume loss. Loss or atrophy of dendritic arborization, neurons, and myelin all occur. Loss of neurons in the thalamus has been estimated to be as great as 35% by the end stage of the disease [4]. If this were representative of the grey matter overall (neglecting contributions from other factors), a loss of 0,55×35%=19% , suggesting an average annual loss of almost 0.5% over 40 years, would be observed.

These calculations are based on imperfect assumptions, but the predicted net annual rate of volume loss (0.1%+0.2%+0.5%+0.4%=1.3%) is in fair agreement with values measured [1, 8-10]. Approximately 100×(0.9%/1.3%)=69%. This leads us to conclude that atrophy measurements – in the absence of significant changes in extracellular water content (see below) – largely reflect axonal (and associated myelin) loss in *normal*-appearing brain tissue of the white and grey matter. Of course, this is undoubtedly an oversimplification. Based on observations in primary neurodegenerative diseases such as Alzheimer's [28], for example, there may be an additional contribution from changes in the extent of dendritic arborization around neuronal soma in grey matter, but this remains to be demonstrated clearly. However, this set of calculations clearly puts the pathology of the macroscopic lesions in a humbler place than they had occupied previously!

Conceptual Problems in the Interpretation of Brain Atrophy

Atrophy Measures Underestimate Axonal Loss in White Matter

While interpretations of brain atrophy measures can reasonably be framed in terms of neuronal and axonal loss, the brain substance also includes a substantial extracellular compartment. Direct histopathological measures [6] confirm an expansion of the extracellular space over the course of the disease. Thus, brain volume change does not provide a direct, quantitative index of axonal loss. Similar observations have been made in a study focusing on the corticospinal tracts in the spinal cord. The area of these tracts and their axon density were reduced at all levels in MS, indicating that axon loss occurs throughout the length of the neuraxis [29]. Measures of white matter volume loss must underestimate the volume loss in the axonal and myelin compartment.

The Substrate for Atrophy in Different Tissue Compartments Varies

Grey matter and white matter make similar contributions to total brain volume. There are differences in the relative contributions from different cell types whose loss could contribute to atrophy in these compartments, however. Myelin loss could make a greater contribution to white matter volume loss than to that of grey matter, for example. Neuronal or dendritic atrophy would make a large contribution to grey matter volume loss specifically.

Neuronal loss clearly occurs in MS. A study combining magnetic resonance techniques and histopathological methods demonstrated that thalamic neurons were reduced by 30%-35%, which accounts for much of the measured thalamic atrophy [4]. Cortical lesions are common in MS [2, 30] and synaptic loss can be prominent within these lesions [31]. Grey matter atrophy contributes to overall atrophy in MS [4, 16, 32]. Grey and white matter also show differential injury at different stages in the disease [33]. This means that the interpretation of atrophy measures may change with the stage of disease.

Brain Atrophy Can Be Regionally Specific, As Well As Confined to Particular Tissue Compartments

One of the most intriguing recent sets of observations has been those showing that MS can affect brain regions differentially. Using a novel technique of automated surface reconstruction, Sailer and colleagues demonstrated a 30% decrease in cortical thickness in MS patients compared to healthy controls [34]. More important is their observation that cortical atrophy follows a distinct pattern in MS patients over time. They used a novel image analysis technique that segmented out the cortex from the brain and removed the confound of gyral folding by inflating the folded cortical surface. This approach allowed highly accurate measurements of not only overall cortical thickness, but also local cortical thickness in different regions. Their study revealed that cortical thinning in MS started in temporal and frontal areas, specifically involving the superior temporal gyrus and superior and middle frontal gyri in the early disease course. Patients with longer disease courses or severe disability exhibited an additional thinning of the motor cortex. Two different mechanisms could underlie this progressive cortical atrophy: one hypothesis is that remote axonal damage could lead to retrograde neuroaxonal degeneration, and the other possibility is that cortical pathology itself could cause cortical atrophy.

Extracellular Water Shifts Can Contribute Significantly to Measures of Volume Change

Although only alluded to briefly above, a final important factor is any change in water content in the extracellular compartment. Acutely, fluid shifts can be major factors accounting for brain volume changes measured by MRI. Dramatic changes have been reported after dialysis (which can be associated with volume decreases of up to 3%) [35], acute dehydration [36], or rehydration after an extended period of malnutrition and alcohol abuse [37, 38].

Inflammatory lesions of MS are associated with increases in water content. Water volume can change rapidly (and can provide part of the contrast mechanism for T_2-hyperintense lesions). Water content can be increased by 10%-20% in the inflammatory lesions of MS [39]. Water content changes also are found in the normal-appearing brain tissue [40]. Short-term changes in brain volume may therefore be accounted for by water content changes rather than "atrophy" arising from myelin loss and neuroaxonal degeneration.

Anti-inflammatory treatment can have substantial effects on water content, complicating the interpretation of brain volume change measurements. High-dose steroids given intravenously for acute exacerbations can decrease brain volume for 2 months following treatment [41]. Therapy with anti-inflammatory drugs such as β-interferons alters brain water content [42]. Not surprisingly, this is associated with decreases in brain volume over the short term [8]. A trial in secondary progressive MS, which did not find any significant effect of treatment on brain after 3 years, observed a similar effect of β-interferon during the first 6 months of treatment, during which a greater reduction of cerebral volume was seen in the interferon than in the control group [21]. This may be a reflection more of a relative loss of oedema than the irreversible loss of axons and myelin. However, all existing immunomodulatory therapies have shown only limited effects on progressive atrophy in the long term [35-38].

Practical Approaches to the Measurement of Brain and White Matter Volume Changes

Here we will discuss techniques for measurement of brain volume changes based on MRI and consider specifically ways in which changes in the white matter compartment can be measured. There is perhaps more information relevant to understanding the substrate for atrophy here. Pathological, imaging, and spectroscopic data confirm that axonal loss is related to local white matter atrophy [5]. The white matter is also a good focus for attention in testing the relation between inflammatory lesions and tissue change as the macroscopic lesions in white matter are well observed by MRI.

There have been a number of approaches to measurement of brain volume change in the white matter. It is important to appreciate these differences to understand why measures made with different approaches cannot be compared directly (although their measurements of change may be correlated) and why sensitivities to change may be different.

Linear Measures of Brain Volume Loss

The most obvious manifestation of white matter volume change is ventriculomegaly. Initial strategies relied upon linear measures of the width of the brain, the corpus callosum, and the third and lateral ventricles [20]. Manual measurements of these regions showed significant volume decreases even over 1 year. The extent of linear measures of change depends on the selected region: larger changes per year were seen in the third ventricle (+4.5%), lateral ventricle width (+5.5%), and corpus callosum (–4.9%), but only smaller changes in brain width (–0.64%). These methods have the advantage of being relatively simple and they can be performed on non-digitized data.

However, the methods are only moderately reproducible, even in the hands of an experienced observer. Uncertainties in the reproducibility of positioning of the linear markers is a concern. For example, in trying to measure the inter-caudate distance from the point of minimum distance may be difficult to define. While objective approaches can be developed, the degree of precision will vary with the extent of atrophy, as with increasing atrophy there is enlargement of the potential areas across which the linear measures can be made. Another concern with these measures is that they rely upon what is effectively a surrogate for the volume change. As the geometry of the ventricles is complex, it must be assumed that all regions expand outward in a simple and highly correlated way – but this cannot be the case in reality. For example, if lesions occur preferentially in the frontal lobes, a relatively greater focal substance loss in the frontal region would be expected.

Semi-manual Estimation of Brain Volume Loss

A first approach to measurement of brain volume change more directly was described by Losseff et al., who defined the large central volume of brain based on anatomical criteria [1]. Using a semi-manual technique, the brain was separated from the skull in each slice of the volume and the aggregate was recorded at each time point. This study detected progressive cerebral atrophy in MS over a course of 18 months. This method has also been applied successfully in large clinical treatment trials [21, 43]. In principle, this approach could have been extended such that, based on signal intensity changes, the white matter volume itself was separately measured at the two time points and its change defined.

An alternative approach is to use the Cavalieri method with stereological point counting [9, 44]. This method overlays a grid system on brain or cervical cord sections, sampling the structure of interest. The number of points covering the structural transects is recorded and volumes are estimated as the sum of the points counted on all transects multiplied by the sectioning interval. Using this technique Edwards and colleagues found more atrophy in secondary progressive than in relapsing-remitting MS [44].

Automated, Whole-Brain Approaches to Volume Measurement

Subsequent approaches have focused on measuring the total brain volume. From measurement of volume at two times, an estimate of atrophy can be made. An advantage of these methods is that they do not suffer from potential bias in selection of the central brain slices. They also are more readily automated – a particular advantage when using large datasets.

The first of these methods was the brain parenchymal volume measurement approach developed by Elizabeth Fisher [8, 18]. In this method the volume of brain is calculated from measurement of the difference in volumes inside a mesh over the exterior surface of the brain and inside the ventricles. A partial volume correction is employed to limit sensitivity to CSF within the sulcal spaces.

This method is highly precise. This has been confirmed in phantom images and by comparing manual outlining with the automatic technique. Results are also highly reproducible across different images from the same brain acquired over a short time period. Differences in the field of interest and segmentation partially cancel out since only one segmentation is performed to obtain the ratio of volume of parenchymal brain tissue to the total volume within the outer surface of the brain. The brain parenchymal fraction (BPF) is then measured from data collected at two time points and percent changes in BPF reflect changes in brain volume. A significant reduction of the BPF was observed in relapsing-remitting MS in a 2-year trial, with a mean BPF change of –1.1% over 2 years (–0.55% p.a.) [8]. A follow-up study of the subsequent 6 years found a lesser annual atrophy rate of –0.33% [18]. A potential disadvantage of this technique is the insensitivity to increases in the external CSF space that will occur with progressive atrophy. Again, in principle this method could be extended by segmentation of white matter within the brain volume to measure its change between the two times.

A similar method has been proposed by Louis Collins at the Montreal Neurological Institute, although it has important differences [45]. With the Brain to IntraCranial Capacity Ratio (BICCR), brain tissue is segmented as a primary step. The segmentation of the brain is explicitly designed to allow segmentation of different tissue types within the brain, leading directly to a measure of white matter. The volume of brain tissue (or that in any compartment) is measured with respect to the volume of the inner table of the skull. By measuring differences in brain volume between times, it provides a measure of brain volume change.

In assessing these and related methods, it is important to consider both accuracy and precision. The accuracy is determined in part by instrument factors, such as the calibration of the gradients and their linearity (which are responsible for the mapping of physical distance into the MR image space). To the extent that the imaging gradients are non-uniform over the brain volume, positioning differences between measurements can reduce accuracy. Accuracy is also determined by the way in which the brain tissue is segmented.

Precision is affected directly by measurement factors but also by the ability of the analysis algorithm to match the brain volumes between two observations.

Direct Measures of Brain Volume Change

The latter problem may be minimized in principle by measurements based directly on measures of volume change. Fox and colleagues measured volume changes over time by subtracting baseline and follow-up scans [10]. The serial scans from an individual are accurately registered and the cerebral volume change may be derived directly. This method measures brain volume changes by integrating the shifts in brain-CSF boundaries caused by cerebral atrophy. The integral called brain boundary shift integral (BBSI) represents the total volume difference between serial scans. This method was used to detect brain atrophy over a 1-year period in definite MS [10] and in patients at the earliest clinical stage of MS [17].

Another and increasingly popular approach to measuring total brain volume change is SIENA (Structural Image Evaluation, using Normalization, of Atrophy) [46]. The method decreases variance in measurements of volume change by estimating directly the local shifts in brain edges rather than average changes in volumes across the entire brain.

The first processing stage is the automated extraction of the brain from the whole-head image using a brain surface mesh which deforms under various smoothness constraints until it fits the brain surface. Secondly, the outer surface of the skull is estimated. The brain volumes at the two time points are then co-registered with the outer table of the skull as a scaling constraint (i.e. it is assumed that the skulls are unchanging and must match perfectly across time) and the transformation mapping one brain into the other is found. Then tissue segmentation is performed to segment the extracted brain into grey matter, white matter, and CSF. The tissue segmentation labels are used to find all brain/non-brain edge points. At each edge point the two (registered) images are compared, in order to find the lateral edge motion between the two time points. Measuring percentage brain volume change (PBVC) with this technique is highly precise and accurate with an error of 0.15% [47]. Like BICCR, an advantage of the approach is that the method is fully automated. However, it should ideally be used with some degree of manual oversight, as (depending on image contrast and brain shape) in some circumstances the brain is not accurately defined, e.g. eyes can be included. Since each brain is matched against itself at another time point, this method potentially has higher precision than methods that measure total brain volume change.

As discussed above, the principle of this type of method can be extended to include selective measures of a specific brain compartment, for example, finding the white matter edges to be used to match these changes specifically. This method has been used successfully to measure cortical atrophy selectively in MS [33]. However, there are a number of complexities in this procedure that should be appreciated to understand the possible sources of error in this type of measurement.

Conclusions

Although the specific focus of this chapter has been on white matter changes, the progressive brain atrophy in MS involves both white and grey matter. It is clear that it occurs at all clinical stages of MS and can be detected from the earliest clinical stage. In the white matter, it develops not only in regions previously affected by inflammatory lesions, but also in the NAWM, where it probably reflects axonal loss induced by Wallerian degeneration.

Care must be taken in comparison of results from different methods, because they measure different parameters – simple estimates of percent change are *not* directly comparable between methods. Measures of whole-brain volume changes may miss regional variations in relative volume loss, an issue that deserves further study.

Interpretation of short-term measures of brain volume changes is complicated by a dependence on water shifts. Without independent measures of relative tissue water content, these cannot be interpreted in a simple way. Nonetheless, because measures of brain atrophy have high precision and can be made from easily acquired (or retrospectively acquired) data, they are important as a measure of pathological outcomes in clinical trials evaluating potential neuroprotective therapies.

Acknowledgements. PMM and SS thank the MRC for support of the Functional Magnetic Resonance Imaging of the Brain Centre. The authors thank the UK Medical Research Council (PMM), the Engineering and Physical Science Research Council (SS) and the EC Marie Curie Programme (CW) for support. They also thank their several colleagues for their generous contribution of expertise and data helpful in generating the ideas presented here, particularly Prof. Nicola de Stefano of the University of Siena.

References

1. Losseff NA, Wang L, Lai HM et al (1996) Progressive cerebral atrophy in multiple sclerosis. A serial MRI study. Brain 119:2009-2019
2. Peterson JW, Bo L, Mork S et al (2001) Transected neurites, apoptotic neurons, and reduced inflammation in cortical multiple sclerosis lesions. Ann Neurol 50:389-400
3. Ferguson B, Matyszak MK, Esiri MM et al (1997) Axonal damage in acute multiple sclerosis lesions. Brain 120:393-399
4. Cifelli A, Arridge M, Jezzard P et al (2002) Thalamic neurodegeneration in multiple sclerosis. Ann Neurol 52:650-653

5. Evangelou N, Konz D, Esiri MM et al (2000) Regional axonal loss in the corpus callosum correlates with cerebral white matter lesion volume and distribution in multiple sclerosis. Brain 123:1845-1849
6. Evangelou N, Esiri MM, Smith S et al (2000) Quantitative pathological evidence for axonal loss in normal appearing white matter in multiple sclerosis. Ann Neurol 47:391-395
7. Coles AJ, Wing MG, Molyneux P et al (1999) Monoclonal antibody treatment exposes three mechanisms underlying the clinical course of multiple sclerosis. Ann Neurol 46:296-304
8. Rudick RA, Fisher E, Lee J-C et al (1999) Use of the brain parenchymal fraction to measure whole brain atrophy in relapsing-remitting MS. Neurology 53:1698-1704
9. Liu C, Edwards S, Gong Q et al (1999) Three dimensional MRI estimates of brain and spinal cord atrophy in multiple sclerosis. J Neurol Neurosurg Psychiatry 66:323-330
10. Fox NC, Jenkins R, Leary SM et al (2000) Progressive cerebral atrophy in MS. A serial study using registered, volumetric MRI. Neurology 54:807-812
11. Coffey CE, Wilkinson WE, Parashos IA et al (1992) Quantitative cerebral anatomy of the aging human brain: a cross-sectional study using magnetic resonance imaging. Neurology 42:527-536
12. Pfefferbaum A, Mathalon DH, Sullivan EV et al (1994) A quantitative magnetic resonance imaging study of changes in brain morphology from infancy to late adulthood. Arch Neurol 51:874-887
13. Gur RC, Mozley PD, Resnick SM et al (1991) Gender differences in age effect on brain atrophy measured by magnetic resonance imaging. Proc Natl Acad Sci USA 88:2845-2849
14. Scahill RI, Frost C, Jenkins R et al (2003) A longitudinal study of brain volume changes in normal aging using serial registered magnetic resonance imaging. Arch Neurol 60:989-994
15. Dalton CM, Brex PA, Jenkins R et al (2002) Progressive ventricular enlargement in patients with clinically isolated syndromes is associated with the early development of multiple sclerosis. J Neurol Neurosurg Psychiatry 73:141-147
16. Chard DT, Griffin CM, Parker GJM et al (2002) Brain atrophy in clinically early relapsing-remitting multiple sclerosis. Brain 125:327-337
17. Brex PA, Jenkins R, Fox NC et al (2000) Detection of ventricular enlargement in patients at the earliest clinical stage of MS. Neurology 54:1689-1691
18. Fisher E, Rudick RA, Simon JH et al (2002) Eight-year follow-up study of brain atrophy in patients with MS. Neurology 59:1412-1420
19. Narayanan S, Fu L, Pioro E et al (1997) Imaging of axonal damage in multiple sclerosis: spatial distribution of magnetic resonance imaging lesions. Ann Neurol 41:385-391
20. Simon JH, Jacobs LD, Campion MK et al (1999) A longitudinal study of brain atrophy in relapsing multiple sclerosis. Neurology 53:139-148
21. Molyneux PD, Kappos L, Polman C et al (2000) The effect of interferon beta-1b treatment on MRI measures of cerebral atrophy in secondary progressive multiple sclerosis. European Study Group on Interferon beta-1b in secondary progressive multiple sclerosis. Brain 123:2256-2263
22. van Walderveen MAA, Kamphorst W, Scheltens P et al (1998) Histopathologic correlate of hypointense lesions on T1-weighted spin-echo MRI in multiple sclerosis. Neurology 50:1282-1288
23. Sailer M, Losseff N, Wang L et al (2001) T1 lesion load and cerebral atrophy as a marker for clinical progression in patients with multiple sclerosis. A prospective 18 months follow-up study. Eur J Neurol 8:37-42
24. Paolillo A, Pozzilli C, Gasperini C et al (2000) Brain atrophy in relapsing-remitting multiple sclerosis: relationship with 'black holes', disease duration and clinical dis-

ability. J Neurol Sci 174:85-91
25. Adams C (1998) A colour atlas of multiple sclerosis and other myelin disorders. Wolfe, London
26. De Stefano N, Iannucci G, Sormani MP et al (2002) MR correlates of cerebral atrophy in patients with multiple sclerosis. J Neurol 249:1072-1077
27. Prineas JW, Connell F (1979) Remyelination in multiple sclerosis. Ann Neurol 5:22-31
28. Uylings HB, de Brabander JM (2002) Neuronal changes in normal human aging and Alzheimer's disease. Brain Cogn 49:268-276
29. DeLuca G, Ebers GC, Esiri MM (2003) Axonal loss in multiple sclerosis: a pathological survey of the corticospinal and sensory tracts [abstract]. Brain Pathol 13:48
30. Bö L, Vedeler CA, Nyland HI et al (2003) Subpial demyelination in the cerebral cortex of multiple sclerosis patients. J Neuropathol Exp Neurol 62:723-732
31. Wegner C, Esiri MM, Palace J et al (2003) Synaptic loss in cortical lesions of multiple sclerosis [abstract]. Mult Scler 9:P612
32. De Stefano N, Matthews PM, Filippi M et al (2003) Evidence of early cortical atrophy in MS: relevance to white matter changes and disability. Neurology 60:1157-1162
33. Chen J, Matthews PM, Arnold DL et al (2001) Regional brain atrophy in multiple sclerosis: increasing sensitivity to differences in relapsing-remitting and secondary-progressive disease [abstract]. Proc Intl Soc Mag Reson Med 9:265
34. Sailer M, Fischl B, Salat D et al (2003) Focal thinning of the cerebral cortex in multiple sclerosis. Brain 126:1734-1744
35. Walters RJ, Fox NC, Crum WR et al (2001) Haemodialysis and cerebral oedema. Nephron 87:143-147
36. Mellanby A, Reveley M (1982) Effects of acute dehydration on computerized tomographic assessment of cerebral density and ventricular volume. Lancet 2:874
37. Carlen P, Wotzmann G, Holgate R et al (1978) Reversible brain atrophy in recently abstinent alcoholics measured by computed tomography scans. Science 200:1076-1078
38. Ron M, Acker W, Shaw G et al (1982) Computerized tomography of the brain in chronic alcoholism: a survey and follow-up study. Brain 105:497-514
39. Helms G (2003) Volume correction for oedema in single-volume proton MR spectroscopy of contrast-enhancing multiple sclerosis lesions. Magn Reson Med 46:256-263
40. Whittall K, MacKay A, Li D et al (2002) Normal-appearing white matter in multiple sclerosis has heterogenous, diffusely prolonged T2. Magn Reson Med 47:403-408
41. Rao AB, Richert N, Howard T et al (2002) Methylprednisolone effect on brain volume and enhancing lesions in MS before and during IFNbeta-1b. Neurology 59:688-694
42. Parry A, Corkill R, Blamire AM et al (2003) Beta-Interferon treatment does not always slow the progression of axonal injury in multiple sclerosis. J Neurol 250:171-178.
43. Stevenson VL, Miller DH, Leary SM et al (2000) One year follow up study of primary and transitional progressive multiple sclerosis. J Neurol Neurosurg Psychiatry 68:713-718
44. Edwards SG, Gong QY, Liu C et al (1999) Infratentorial atrophy on magnetic resonance imaging and disability in multiple sclerosis. Brain 122:291-301
45. Collins DL, Montagnat J, Zijdenbos A et al (2001) Automated estimation of brain volume in multiple sclerosis with BICCR. Lect Notes Comput Sci 2082:141-147
46. Smith SM, De Stefano N, Jenkinson M et al (2001) Normalized accurate measurement of longitudinal brain change. J Comput Assist Tomogr 25:466-475
47. Smith SM, Zhang Y, Jenkinson M et al (2002) Accurate, robust, and automated longitudinal and cross-sectional brain change analysis. Neuroimage 17:479-489

Chapter 4

Normal-Appearing White Matter Changes in Multiple Sclerosis: Magnetization Transfer

F. Fazekas, C. Enzinger, S. Ropele

Introduction and Background

Magnetization exchange is a physicochemical mechanism which generally occurs between protons within a tissue. With appropriate techniques this mechanism can be used to augment tissue contrast and, even more importantly, to explore specific tissue characteristics [1]. One such approach is to saturate only a certain proton species and thereby to determine its contribution to a given tissue from the observed signal reduction, commonly known as "saturation transfer". This is understood best when biological tissue is considered as consisting of at least two kinds of protons that differ in their molecular mobility, i.e. a pool of motionally restricted protons – those bound to macromolecules such as myelin proteins and lipids of brain tissue – and another pool of freely mobile protons in tissue water. The different mobility of these protons is reflected by different transverse relaxation times and hence by different spectral line widths. The free water protons with little spin-spin interaction have a very narrow spectral line width. In contrast, macromolecular protons, due to their diverse interactions, have a very broad line width which can be up to 100 kHz (Fig. 1). If a train of short radiofrequency (RF) saturation pulses is applied with a RF offset and band width that partly matches the shape of the absorption line of the macromolecular protons, these macromolecular protons will become saturated. By various mechanisms this saturation is partly transferred to the "MR-visible" water protons, thus "magnetization transfer" (MT). Therefore, a reduction of overall signal intensity occurs if such saturation pulses are applied prior to a conventional imaging sequence (Fig. 1). This effect can be quantified in a relative manner by calculation of the magnetization transfer ratio (MTR). This ratio indicates the percentage difference in signal intensities between images acquired with and without prior RF saturation of the macromolecular proton pool. This is expressed as follows:

$$\mathrm{MTR}=[S_0-S_s/S_0]\times 100\%$$

where S_0 is signal without and S_s signal with saturation of the macromolecular pool. The MTR is mainly a function of the magnetization exchange kinetics and of the intrinsic longitudinal relaxation time of the water protons. Clearly, as a larger macromolecular pool will make the exchange mechanism more efficient, the MTR also depends on the macromolecular density. It is important to note

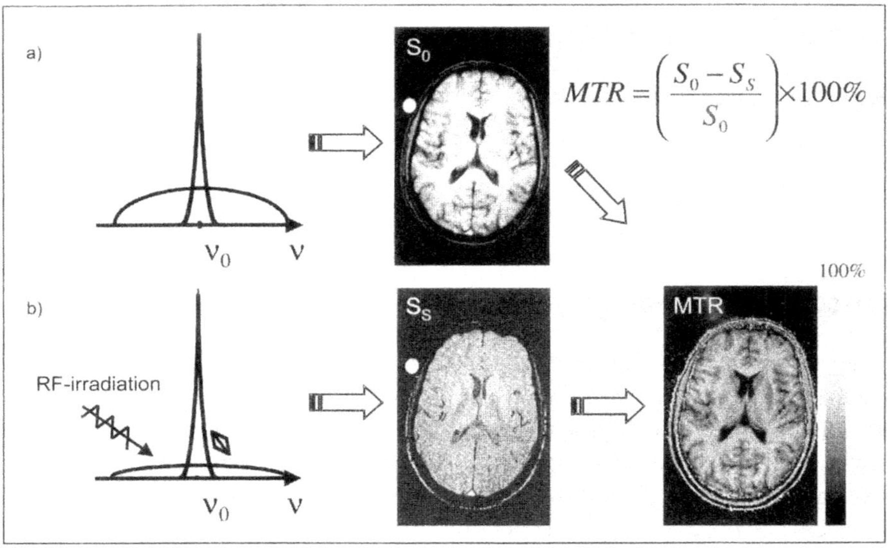

Fig. 1a, b. Magnetization transfer (MT) process and its consequences on the signal obtained from different brain tissues. The bound (macromolecular) protons with their wide spectral line width (as shown in a) are saturated in **b**. Note the resulting signal reduction (compared to **a**), which is much more obvious in white matter than in grey matter structures. The relative signal differences between **a** and **b** are reflected in the MTR map

that the MTR also strongly depends on the pulse sequence design and, in particular, on the RF characteristics of the saturation pulses in terms of flip angle, duration, resonance offset, and duty cycle.

In terms of imaging results, the observed signal from a given tissue decreases as the proportion of bound protons increases, i.e. a larger magnetization transfer effect. Therefore brain tissue becomes darker after pre-saturation of the macromolecular pool, which is especially pronounced for white matter regions. Inversely, this translates into a higher MTR (Fig. 1).

Clearly, the MTR gives only a semi-quantitative measure of the MT phenomenon, as pulse sequence design and various relaxation properties will also contribute to the MTR. A more comprehensive analysis of the MT and relaxation mechanism would also include the exchange rates, relative pool sizes, and native transverse and longitudinal relaxation rates of the macromolecular and water protons [2]. Such approaches are addressed below. Independent of these more sophisticated considerations, however, even the rather crude approach of determining the differences in MT effects by calculating the MTR has already provided significant insights in multiple sclerosis (MS) (for a recent review see [3]). This can be attributed to several factors. First, the proportion of bound protons in white matter is especially high and, as a consequence, changes in the composition of white matter readily impact on the MT process. Second, even as a relative measure the MTR allows quantitative deductions about the composition of tissue to a certain extent. Furthermore, it has been shown that the MTR values can be very reproducible and comparable among subjects when using similar data acquisition schemes and appropriate technical corrections [4].

Along these lines, MT imaging has been successfully used to describe the severity of tissue damage in MS lesions in both a cross-sectional and a longitudinal manner. It was observed that the MTR drops dramatically when MS lesions start to enhance, and that it can show partial or even complete recovery in the subsequent 1-6 months [5-7]. As such rapid changes cannot be explained by oedema alone, this dynamics is thought to result primarily from demyelination and remyelination. Hence, MT changes are frequently seen as an ideal means of monitoring this important pathological process in MS. Evidence for this assumption also comes from the comparison of MTR values with other MR metrics known to reflect the severity of brain tissue damage, such as the so-called "black holes" on T1-weighted scans. MTR was found to correlate inversely with the degree of hypointensity and MTR was seen to increase when MS lesions changed from T1 hypointensity to T1 isointensity [7]. Histopathologically this return to isointensity of lesions was shown to correlate with remyelination, whereas persistent hypointensity was found in demyelinated lesions [8].

The possibility of applying techniques like the calculation of tissue-based histograms to the analysis of MT effects has contributed greatly to the utility of this method [9]. With this highly automated technique, it is possible to evaluate large tissue classes within the entire brain in terms of MT behaviour. Several histogram metrics have been shown to differ between MS patients and controls. MS patients typically have lower average MTR histogram peak height and position, which indicates that essentially the entire brain is affected by the disease [10].

MT and Normal-Appearing White Matter

Given the robustness of MTR measurements and the possibility of detecting abnormalities not seen by conventional MRI, researchers started to look not only at the changes in MS lesions but also set out to evaluate the white matter which appears normal on conventional scans (normal-appearing white matter; NAWM). Filippi et al. were among the first to note that NAWM close to MS lesions has a reduced MTR [11]. This was especially the case in patients with secondary progressive MS (SPMS). The aetiology of this MTR reduction can be manifold. The observation that NAWM MTR abnormalities are more likely and more pronounced with advanced disease suggests secondary phenomena such as axonal destruction by Wallerian degeneration and gliosis. On the other hand, there is quite firm evidence that MTR changes precede lesion formation in NAWM. Various researchers have demonstrated MTR reductions in the NAWM as long as 2 years before lesion formation [12-14]. Oedema, marked astrocytic proliferation, perivascular inflammation, demyelination, and axonal loss may all account for an increased amount of unbound water in the NAWM and consequently provoke these MTR changes.

Further attempts have been made recently to identify and characterize the different components contributing to the overall MT effect more precisely. This assessment of individual parameters of the MT process is generally in agreement with previous MTR studies [15]. In addition, a longitudinal analysis of 12 MS patients for up to 1 year using a Fast-PACE (Phase Acquisition of Composite Echoes) sequence showed that the appearance of new active lesions was preceded by a significant decrease not only of the MTR but also of the magnetization forward transfer rate (k_{for}) and by an increase of T_{1free} [16] (Fig. 2). The drop of k_{for} was the most pronounced pre-lesional change and together with the MTR was statistically significant as early as 4 months before the appearance of new lesions. The observed increase of T_{1free} was relatively small and occurred only closer to new lesion appearance. Thus the pool of bound protons appears to diminish before there is evidence for blood-brain barrier leakage as indicated by an increase of T_{1free}. This constellation would suggest that some kind of damage to myelin is among the leading events in lesion formation, and supports the notion that demyelination might occur even prior to or at least partly independent from overt and acute inflammatory events. Unfortunately, the sensitivity of this technique is not yet sufficiently high to reliably identify in advance areas of NAWM exhibiting changes in tissue composition that, while subtle, are pronounced enough to give rise to or serve as a focus for a new lesion later on. We therefore also do not know whether these changes are potentially reversible and what thresholds have to be exceeded on the way to the formation of lesions visible on conventional MRI. So far, evidence of pre-lesional changes can only be obtained in retrospect, i.e. by looking back at preceding MT changes at the location of a now apparent new lesion, and by the pooling of information from a large number of lesions. Despite this drawback, information about disease-related changes in the MT process obtained in a more complex manner such as that provided by multiparametric analysis obviously helps us to gain additional insights into the pathophysiology of lesion formation in MS.

Information on NAWM in MS from MT histogram analyses usually comes from studies on normal-appearing whole-brain tissue (NABT), i.e. from histograms which include grey matter structures. This is nonetheless reasonable because the MTR of grey matter is normally much lower. As a consequence, most NABT histogram metrics are governed primarily by the composition of white matter. Primary progressive (PP) MS patients were shown to have a significantly lower histogram peak height with a normal peak position and only a slightly reduced average MTR, which would be in line with the presence of subtle but widespread damage to the NAWM [17, 18]. Patients with relapsing-remitting (RR) MS had both a lower average MTR and a lower peak height than healthy controls, and these differences were even more pronounced in patients with SPMS [19, 20]. The importance of these observations comes from the fact that they indicate the presence of more diffuse damage to the brain white matter than

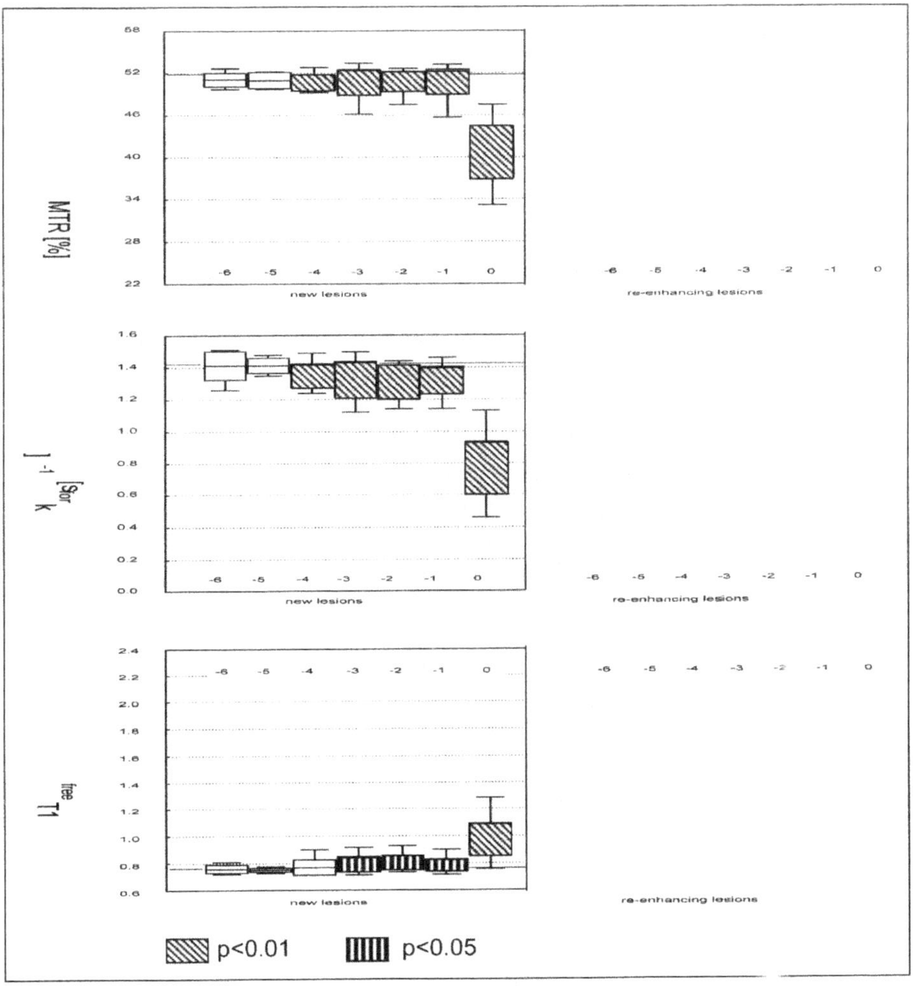

Fig. 2. MT parameters from pre-lesional NAWM over a period of 6 months before the appearance of a new enhancing lesion. a Magnetization transfer ratio (MTR), b magnetization exchange rate k_{for}, and c T_{1free}. Month 0 is the time of first enhancement. *Bars* represent the range of minimum and maximum values; *boxes* represent the standard deviation and the mean value is indicated by the *line*. The *long horizontal line* represents the mean value of control NAWM. Note that the drop of k_{for} is the most pronounced pre-lesional change and together with the MTR precedes the increase of T_{1free}. (Modified from [16])

one would assume from the observation of disseminated focal MS lesions. In this context, it would be especially interesting to know more about the causality between and the temporal sequence of these events, i.e. whether such diffuse abnormalities are associated with focal lesions or occur independently, and also whether they had preceded MS plaques or were a consequence of them. The reported MT changes in PPMS despite the known paucity of white matter lesions on conventional MRI in this patient group argue strongly for an independent phenomenon. What additional role grey matter pathology may play in this scenario is still difficult to appreciate. On the other hand, in RRMS and SPMS, at least some association between NAWM changes and focal damage can be assumed because of probable distant effects in the perifocal white matter due to axonal damage and transection.

As to the time when NAWM MTR abnormalities may first be observed in the evolution of MS, the data are still contradictory. While some researchers found MTR reductions even at the earliest onset of symptomatic MS such as in clinically isolated syndromes [21], other groups did not confirm this finding [22, 23]. Although differences in patient selection and in the timing of the examinations cannot be ruled out as possible confounding factors, this could also simply reflect differences in the sensitivity of the imaging techniques used to detect MT changes [24]. Interestingly, some reduction in NABT MTR has been reported even in asymptomatic relatives of patients with MS by some investigators [25].

Besides these insights into the pathophysiology of MS, the notion of diffuse damage to the NAWM by MT imaging also helps us to understand in part the "clinico-radiological paradox", that is, the often striking discrepancy between the amount of visible MS lesions and the level of disability of the patients. While various other factors like lesion location, lesion severity, spinal cord damage, etc. are also contributing factors, the role of NAWM cannot be dismissed, especially because it constitutes a large proportion of the brain of MS patients. Diffuse white matter changes may be also especially relevant for MS symptoms that probably originate from a complex disturbance of networks in the brain, such as cognitive problems and fatigue.

Future Prospects

The use of the MT effects to characterize MS-related tissue changes has provided a plethora of new insights into both lesion development and the existence of abnormalities in otherwise normal-appearing brain tissue. Further research will have to aim at determining the earliest occurrence of these abnormalities and their aetiology. In terms of data collection, this demands especially the investigation of large samples of individuals with a clinically isolated syndrome and also of potentially susceptible individuals, such as patients from families with a known high prevalence of MS. The use of similar imaging protocols and standardized physical and mathematical approaches for data correction and normalization may help to satisfy the urgent need for pooling of MTR data from various institutions [4]. Long-term follow-up of patients with a first clinically isolated syndrome suggestive of MS may also clarify the predictive value of MTI changes regarding patient prognosis and could potentially contribute to identifying specific MS subgroups in correspondence to suggestions based on immunopathological data [26].

For these purposes, even more robust and sensitive measurement techniques of the MT effect would be desirable. Advances have been made regarding the quantitation of several fundamental parameters which contribute to the MT exchange. These parameters reflect true biochemical properties and should be less susceptible to the influence of apparatus and sequence parameters than the MTR. So far, different approaches have already been suggested for the estimation of the fundamental in vivo MT parameters. They also appear now to be becoming accessible in time periods which are tolerable for the patient [15, 27, 28].

Finally, to further augment insights into the pathophysiology of MS and to detect treatment effects which would otherwise go unnoticed, increasing use of MT metrics in the evaluation and follow-up of MS patients as well as in MS treatment trials should be encouraged. In the latter regard, the MT results of the European Study on IVIG (intravenous immunoglobulin) in MS (ESIMS) appear of great interest [29]. Over 2 years, the placebo-treated group of patients showed a significant drop of the NABT MTR peak height, whereas no pronounced change over time was observed following IVIG treatment. Although this was not associated with any observable clinical benefit, in extension of the reasoning presented above, this finding allows us to speculate about a protective effect of IVIG on NAWM. However, from the comparison with MTR measurements in another trial in SPMS [30] it also becomes clear that increased efforts will have to be made in the future to assure good reproducibility and comparability of MTI data collected at different centres, and that some consensus will have to be developed regarding their analysis.

Conclusions

MRI techniques using MT effects to characterize brain tissue have provided significant insights into changes of white matter in MS that appears normal on conventional MRI. Further progress may be expected by strategies to define not only the MTR but also the fundamental in vivo MT parameters. In addition to the provision of pathophysiological and clinical insights, NAWM MTI also promises to be very useful in determining and understanding the treatment effects of available and newly developed MS drugs.

Acknowledgements. Stefan Ropele and Christian Enzinger are supported by the FWF Austrian Science Fund, grant numbers P15158 and J2373, respectively.

References

1. Wolff S, Balaban R (1994) Magnetization transfer imaging:practical aspects and clinical applications. Radiology 192:593-599
2. Sled J, Pike G (2001) Quantitative imaging of magnetization transfer exchange and relaxation properties in vivo using MRI. Mag Reson Med 46:923-931

3. Filippi M (2003) Magnetization transfer MRI in multiple sclerosis and other central nervous system disorders. Eur J Neurol 10:3-10
4. Ropele S, Filippi M, Valsasina P et al (2003) Assessment and correction of B1-induced errors in multicentre magnetization transfer studies [Abstract]. Mult Scler 9 (Suppl 1):S 60
5. Dousset V, Gayou A, Brochet B, Caillé JM (1998) Early structural changes in acute MS lesions assessed by serial magnetization transfer studies. Neurology 51:1150-1155
6. Filippi M, Rocca MA, Comi G (1998) Magnetization transfer ratios of multiple sclerosis lesions with variable durations of enhancement. J Neurol Sci 159:162-165
7. van Waesberghe JH, van Walderveen MA, Castelijns JA et al (1998) Patterns of lesion development in multiple sclerosis: longitudinal observations with T1-weighted spin-echo and magnetization transfer MR. AJNR Am J Neuroradiol 19:675-683
8. Bitsch A, Kuhlmann T, Stadelmann C et al (2001) A longitudinal MRI study of histopathologically defined hypointense multiple sclerosis lesions. Ann Neurol 49:793-796
9. van Buchem M, McGowan JC, Lokcon DL et al (1996) Quantitative volumetric magnetization transfer analysis in multiple sclerosis: estimation of macroscopic and microscopic disease burden. Magn Reson Med 36:632-636
10. Filippi M, Grossman RI, Comi G (eds) (1999) Magnetization transfer imaging in multiple sclerosis. Neurology 53(Suppl 3)
11. Filippi M, Campi A, Dousset V et al (1995) A magnetisation transfer imaging study of normal-appearing white matter in multiple sclerosis. Neurology 45:478-482
12. Filippi M, Rocca MA, Martino G et al (1998) Magnetization transfer changes in the normal appearing white matter precede the appearance of enhancing lesions in patients with multiple sclerosis. Ann Neurol 43:809-814
13. Goodkin D, Rooney WD, Sloan R et al (1998) A serial study of new MS lesions and the white matter from which they arise. Neurology 51:1689-1697
14. Pike GB, De Stefano N, Narayanan S et al (2000) Multiple sclerosis: magnetization transfer MR imaging of white matter before lesion appearance on T2-weighted images. Radiology 215:824-830
15. Ropele S, Strasser-Fuchs S, Augustin M et al (2000) A comparison of magnetization transfer ratio, magnetization transfer rate, and the native relaxation time of water protons related to relapsing-remitting multiple sclerosis. AJNR Am J Neuroradiol 21:1885-1891
16. Fazekas F, Ropele S, Enziger C et al (2002) Quantitative magnetization transfer imaging of pre-lesional white-matter changes in multiple sclerosis. Mult Scler 8:479-484
17. Filippi M, Iannucci G, Tortorella C et al (1999) Comparison of MS clinical phenotypes using conventional and magnetization transfer MRI. Neurology 52:588-594
18. Rovaris M, Bozzali M, Santuccio G et al (2001) In vivo assessment of the brain and cervical cord pathology of patients with primary progressive multiple sclerosis. Brain 124:2540-2549
19. Filippi M, Inglese M, Rovaris M et al (2000) Magnetization transfer imaging to monitor the evolution of MS: a 1-year follow-up study. Neurology 55:940-946
20. Kalkers N, Hintzen RQ, van Waesberghe JH et al (2001) Magnetization transfer histogram parameters reflect all dimensions of MS pathology, including atrophy. J Neurol Sci 184:155-162
21. Iannucci G, Tortorella C, Rovaris M et al (2000) Prognostic value of MR and magnetization transfer imaging findings in patients with clinically isolated syndromes suggestive of multiple sclerosis at presentation. AJNR Am J Neuroradiol 21:1034-1038
22. Kaiser J, Grossman RI, Polansky M et al (2000) Magnetization transfer histogram analysis of monosymptomatic episodes of neurologic dysfunction: preliminary findings. AJNR Am J Neuroradiol 21:1043-1047

23. Brex P, Leary SM, Plant GT et al (2001) Magnetization transfer imaging in patients with clinically isolated syndromes suggestive of multiple sclerosis. AJNR Am J Neuroradiol 22:947-951
24. Traboulsee A, Dehmeshki J, Brex PA et al (2002) Normal-appearing brain tissue MTR histograms in clinically isolated syndromes suggestive of MS. Neurology 59:126-128
25. Siger-Zajdel M, Filippi M, Selmaj K (2002) MTR discloses subtle changes in the normal-appearing tissue from relatives of patients with MS. Neurology 58:317-320
26. Lassmann H (2001) Classification of demyelinating diseases at the interface between etiology and pathogenesis. Curr Opin Neurol 14:253-258
27. Ropele S, Stollberger R, Hartung HP, Fazekas F (2000) Estimation of magnetization transfer rates from PACE experiments with pulsed RF saturation. J Magn Reson Imaging 12:749-756
28. Ramani A, Dalton C, Miller DH et al (2002) Precise estimate of fundamental in-vivo MT parameters in human brain in clinically feasible times. Magn Reson Imaging 20:721-731
29. Filippi M, Rocca MA, Pagani E et al (2004) European Study on Intravenous Immunoglobulin in Multiple Sclerosis (ESIMS). Results of magnetization transfer MRI analysis. Arch Neurol (in press)
30. Inglese M, van Waesberghe JH, Rovaris M et al (2003) The effect of interferon beta-1b on quantities derived from MT MRI in secondary progressive MS. Neurology 60:853-860

Chapter 5

The Short T_2 Component in Normal-Appearing White Matter in Multiple Sclerosis

A. MacKay, C. Laule, I. Vavasour, B. Mädler, A. Traboulsee, D. Paty, W. Moore, D. Li

While proton density/T_2-weighted (PD/T2) MR images are exquisitely sensitive to pathology in brain tissue and play a key role in clinical applications of MRI to multiple sclerosis (MS), they are notoriously non-specific for particular brain pathologies. Moreover, the subtle tissue changes which occur in normal-appearing white matter (NAWM) in MS are not visible on PD/T_2 images. However, measurements of T_2 relaxation have the potential to provide more specific information about MS tissue pathology, both in lesions and in NAWM.

T_2 Decay Curves from Brain

T_2-weighted images show tissue contrast at a single TE time, while the T_2 decay curve is a plot of the NMR signal for a wide range of echo times (TE). For a homogeneous sample, the T_2 decay curve is initially (i.e. at TE=0) proportional to proton density and then decays to zero with a single characteristic time constant known as T_2. Pure water at 37 °C has a T_2 of approximately 3 s, while the NMR signal of ice decays to zero in about 10 μs; hence, the T_2 of water is sensitive to its physical state. In brain, the T_2 of water is affected by interactions between water and non-aqueous tissue, and also by diffusion. The T_2 of water in brain can range from several milliseconds to over 1 s, depending upon local tissue microstructure. NMR signals from non-aqueous brain tissue, excluding mobile lipids, decay to zero in much less than 1 ms [1] and consequently are not visible on a clinical MRI scanner.

T_2 decay curve measurement in brain is most conveniently obtained from a multi-echo MR sequence in which the signal is refocused at multiple times during one acquisition. This usually involves application of a slice-selective 90° pulse followed by multiple 180° pulses. For small in vitro samples, it is relatively simple to acquire high-fidelity T_2 decay curves using an NMR spectrometer. The situation in vivo is much more challenging [2, 3]. Despite reproducible T_2 analyses [3, 4], few in vivo T_2 studies have accurately characterized the complete relaxation decay curve from brain.

An MR pulse sequence for quantitative in vivo T_2 measurement must satisfy at least two criteria. Firstly, the 180° pulses must refocus all the magnetization in the selected slice; otherwise estimated T_2 times depend upon the sequence echo spacing. Secondly, a sufficient number of echo times (appropriate spacing and range) must be sampled to adequately characterize the observed decay;

otherwise the estimated T_2 times have little direct relevance to the system being investigated. The multi-echo pulse sequence we use employs a slice-selective 90° pulse, followed by a train of rectangular 180° pulses. A series of slice-select crusher gradient pulses of alternating sign and decreasing amplitude are applied on either side of each 180° pulse. This pulse sequence causes dephasing of flow effects and eliminates signal generated from outside the selected slice [2]. In some circumstances, for example, in the presence of paramagnetic or ferromagnetic constituents (e.g. ferritin), the T_2 decay curve shape depends upon the length of time between successive 180° pulses, or echo spacing [4, 5]. Therefore, for detailed comparison between T_2 studies, results should be acquired with the same echo spacing. These effects are likely to be most pronounced in grey matter structures, such as the globus pallidus, which have relatively high iron content [6].

For a homogeneous system, such as water in a beaker, all hydrogen nuclei are equivalent and the decay curve, $S(t)$, is well fit by a simple decaying exponential function:

$$S(t)=S(0)e^{-\mathrm{TE}/\mathrm{T}_2}.$$

For such a system, a plot of log($S(t)$) vs TE time yields a straight line with slope $-1/T_2$.

Figure 1 shows T_2 decay curves measured from pure water, and from normal white matter, normal grey matter, and an MS lesion in brain. The decay curve from pure water is mono-exponential and follows a straight line on the semi-log-

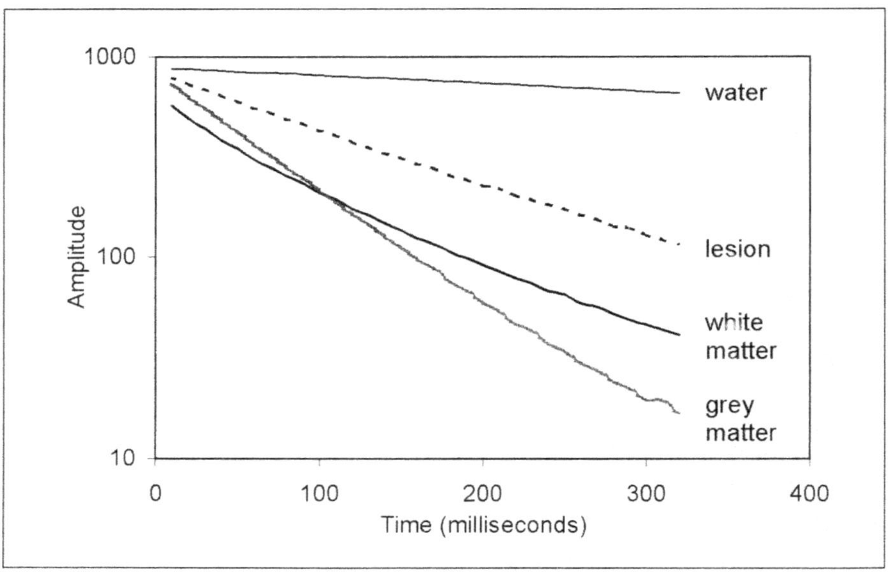

Fig. 1. T_2 decay curves from pure water, an MS lesion, normal white matter, and normal grey matter

arithmic plot, while decay curves from brain cannot be fitted properly by a single straight line, suggesting the existence of more than one water reservoir, each with its own T_2 time. White and grey matter decay curves follow different trajectories for different brain structures. Furthermore, different types of brain pathologies give rise to different decay curves. Since the T_2 decay curve from water in brain is influenced by the local water environment, with appropriate analysis, T_2 decay curves should serve as probes of subvoxel brain structure and consequently provide specific information on brain pathology.

Analysis of T_2 Decay Curves from Brain

T_2 decay curves from brain can be interpreted as sums of exponentials where each exponential component corresponds to a distinguishable water compartment. Extracting exponential relaxation times and amplitudes from in vivo decay curves requires an analysis of the T_2 decay curve to solve for the relative contributions from the various T_2 components:

$$S(t)=\Sigma\, I_i\, e^{-TE/T_{2i}} \text{ (discrete) or } S(t)=\int A(T_2)\, e^{-t/T_2}\, dT_2 \text{ (continuous)},$$

where I_i is proportional to the number of protons with relaxation time T_{2i} and $A(T_2)$ is proportional to the number of protons with relaxation time T_2. $A(T_2)$, known as the T_2 distribution, is the output of the T_2 decay curve analysis. The most common technique for extracting $A(T_2)$ from the decay curve is the non-negative least squares algorithm (NNLS) [7]. Non-negativity is a reasonable physical constraint because there cannot be a negative number of protons contributing to the MR signal. This algorithm is able to construct solutions, $A(T_2)$, ranging from discrete components to smooth distributions. Due to the inhomogeneity of water locations in brain, a smooth solution is most appropriate for T_2 distributions from brain.

Figure 2 shows a smooth NNLS T_2 distribution from a brain volume. Each peak corresponds to a distinguishable water reservoir and its area is proportional to the number of contributing water molecules. T_2 distributions from brain may have several peaks. We [8, 9] assigned, in agreement with others [10-12], the short T_2 component at about 20 ms to water associated with myelin, the peak(s) at 80-100 ms to intra- and extracellular water, and the peak at approximately 2 s to cerebrospinal fluid. The sum of intensities of all the individual T_2 components is proportional to the total amount of water in the chosen volume. Therefore, if the component assignments are correct, we can extract at least two important quantities from T_2 decay curve analysis: (1) the local brain water content and (2) the amount of brain water associated with myelin. The latter should reflect myelin content and promises to provide new understanding about the role of myelin in many neurological disorders.

The myelin water fraction (MWF) is defined as the ratio of the signal with T_2 below 50 ms to the total area of the T_2 distribution. Water in myelin is expected to be, on average, about one-sixth of the total water in white matter [12]; our

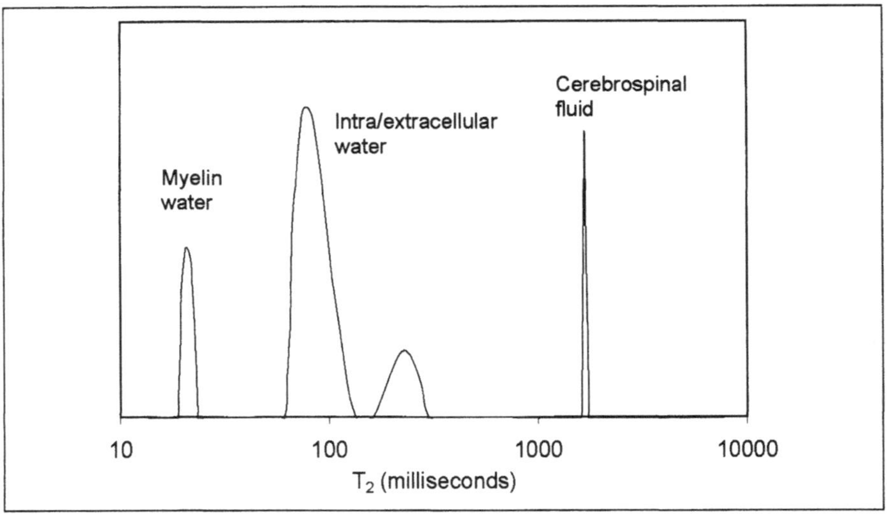

Fig. 2. T_2 distribution from brain. Three different water environments can be separated: myelin water (short T_2 component), intra-/extracellular water, and cerebrospinal fluid

average MWF in white matter of 0.11 is in approximate agreement. Myelin water fractions vary between different brain structures; values for the posterior internal capsules are typically more than twice those from the minor forceps. We believe that this variation arises from differing myelin contents. An image of the MWF may be displayed as a "myelin water map" where regions of white matter, which has high myelin content, appear bright (Fig. 3.).

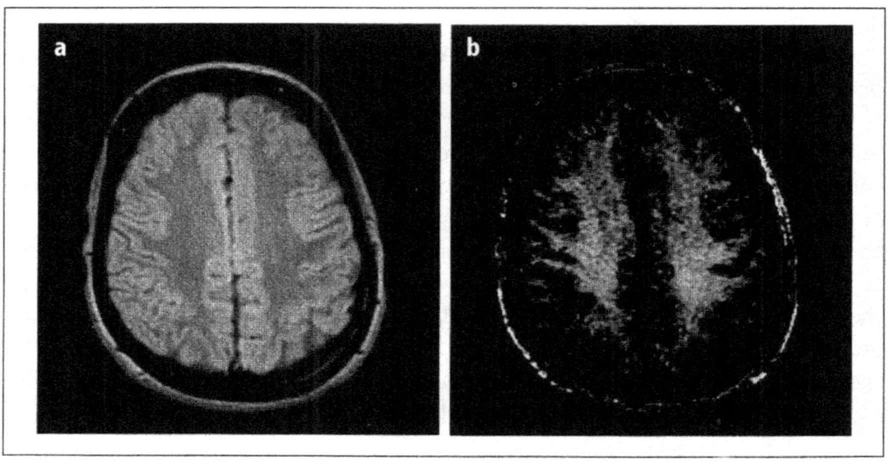

Fig. 3. **a** Conventional proton density MR image and **b** corresponding myelin water map from a normal volunteer. Intensities in the images scale with water content and myelin water fraction, respectively

Comparison to Other Techniques Commonly Used to Explore Brain Pathology

Many investigators have used the magnetization transfer ratio (MTR) as a specific measure of brain pathology [13, 14]. In a primate model [15], it was shown that a lower MTR was associated with demyelination. The MTR value has been found in many studies to be a robust and sensitive indicator of white matter pathology, although it is known to be influenced by water content changes [16, 17]. It is also relatively easy to acquire in a multi-slice imaging study. This has encouraged some groups to envisage the MTR as a specific measure for myelination. If this is true, and if the MWF is also related to myelination, then these two MR quantities should be correlated. Figure 4 shows that for a large of number of sites in normal white matter, MTR and MWF were not highly correlated with each other (R^2=0.05) [18]. Similar results were demonstrated for multiple sclerosis lesions [19]. Therefore, MT and T_2 provide different, yet complementary, information about brain tissue.

In white matter, it has been demonstrated that the apparent diffusion coefficient, *D*, is larger along neurons than it is perpendicular to them [20-22], and therefore *D* must be handled as a tensor, **D**. White matter diffusion anisotropy can be characterized by various parameters derived from the 3×3 diffusion tensor, **D**. A convenient measure which is specifically sensitive to white matter nerve fibre tracts is the fractional anisotropy (FA), which is proportional to the ratio of the standard deviation of the diffusion tensor to its mean principal value. When water diffusion is isotropic, as in pure water, the three principal components of **D** are equal and the FA is zero. For water associated with nerve fibres in white matter, diffusion is much larger along the axon and the FA is large. Since axons are wrapped in myelin, the diffusion FA should be correlated with myelin content

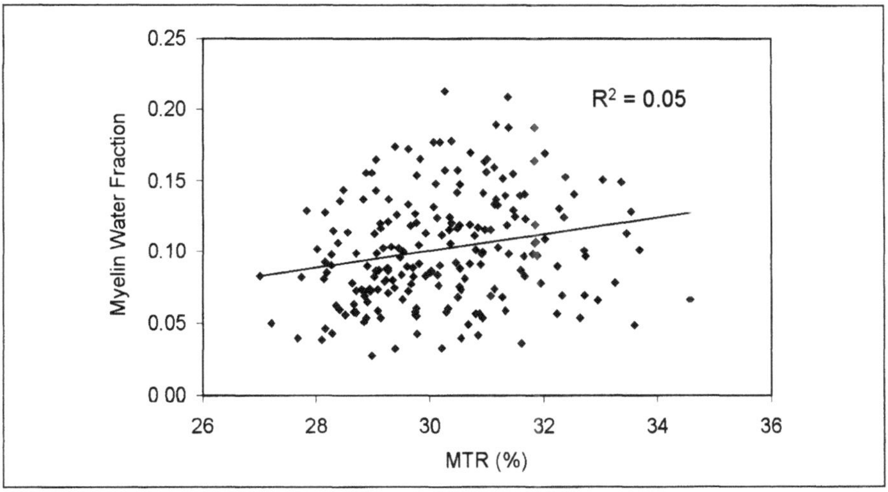

Fig. 4. Relation between magnetization transfer ratio (MTR) and myelin water fraction in white matter. The poor correlation is quantified by the low R^2 (0.05), a measure of the variance in myelin water fraction accounted for by MTR

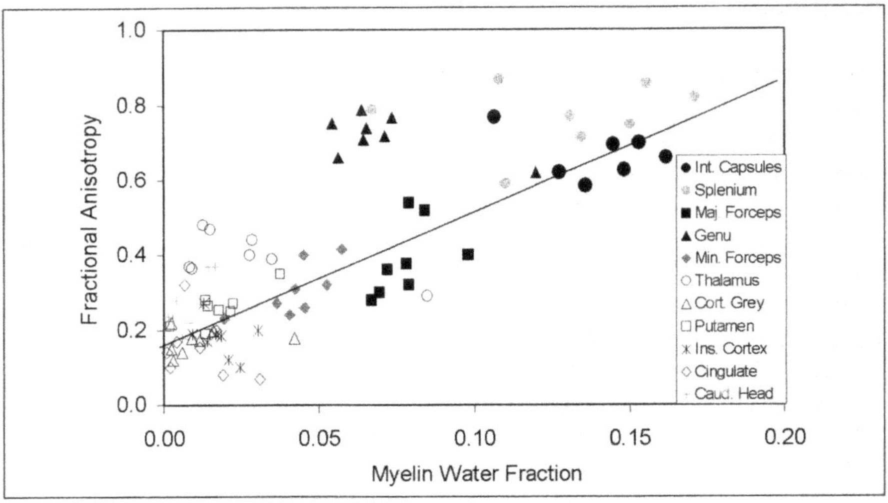

Fig. 5. Relation of diffusion fractional anisotropy with myelin water fraction. A good correlation is seen (R^2=0.6), although specific brain regions systematically fall outside the linear relationship

and therefore also with MWF. Indeed, a significant correlation (R^2=0.6) has been shown between MWF and FA [23] in normal white matter, as demonstrated in Fig. 5, although specific brain structures systematically fall outside the linear relationship. Therefore, diffusion FA and MWF provide similar, but complementary, information about myelinated axons in brain but each probably originates from a different microscopic structure – myelin sheaths in the case of MWF and the axons they ensheath in the case of diffusion FA.

Validation of the MWF Measurement

If the MWF is a marker for myelin, it should correlate with histopathological measurements of myelin. Studies on guinea pig [16, 17] and rat [24] models found the white matter T_2 distributions to be multi-component and found the short T_2 component to be correlated with histological measures of myelin. Fortuitously, the T_2 distribution from formalin-fixed human brain is shaped similarly to that from brain in vivo, although the T_2 times are shifted to shorter times. This is perhaps not surprising since water T_2 times are strongly influenced by cellular structure [25], which is relatively unchanged by fixation. Histopathological studies have shown that the MWF qualitatively corresponds to the anatomic distribution of myelin as demarked by the luxol fast blue stain [26]. Figure 6 [27] shows a strong correlation (R^2=0.81) between MWF and blue optical density in fixed brain slices stained by the luxol fast blue stain for myelin. These studies provide strong evidence that the MWF is a marker for myelin in white matter.

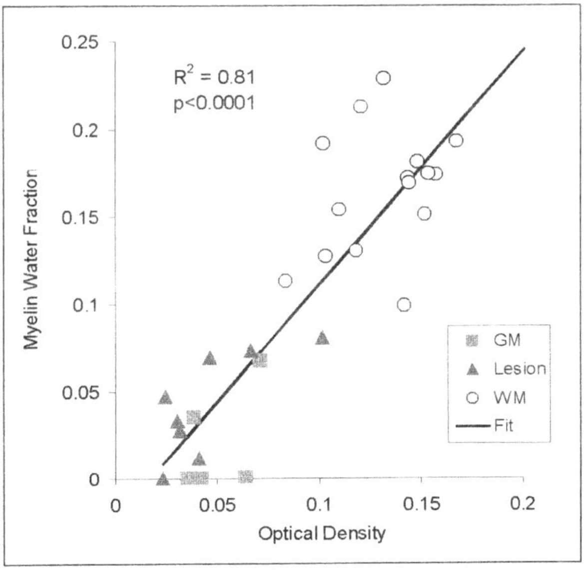

Fig. 6. Example of strong correlation between myelin water fraction and blue optical density of luxol fast blue stain for various regions of interest in a formalin fixed multiple sclerosis brain. (From [27], by permission)

Short T_2 Component Measurements in Multiple Sclerosis Patients

T_2 measurements may have the potential to distinguish the relative roles of oedema, inflammation, myelin loss, axonal loss, and gliosis which occur in MS. In Fig. 7, a myelin water map acquired from an MS patient shows substantially reduced myelin

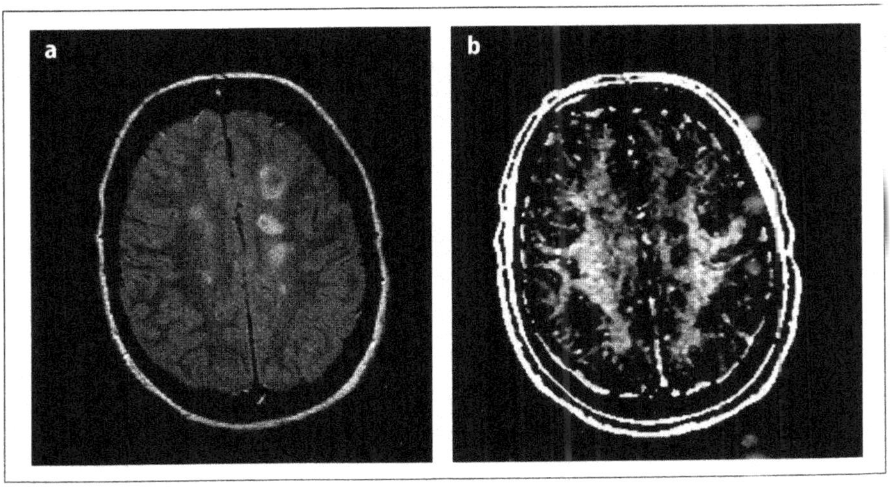

Fig. 7. **a** Conventional proton density MR image and **b** myelin water map for a patient with MS. Lesions show a reduction in myelin and there is a diffuse loss of myelin water in normal-appearing white matter (NAWM)

water in lesions and slightly reduced myelin water in NAWM regions. Comparison of the water content (proton density) and myelin water maps also shows a large region in NAWM which has substantially reduced myelin water. This implies that NAWM pathology may be inhomogeneously distributed throughout the brain.

We recently reported on a study [28] of water content and MWF from NAWM in 33 MS patients and normal white matter (NWM) in 18 age- and gender-matched controls. Of the MS patients (mean age 41 years; range 30-56 years), 24 had a relapsing remitting (RR) disease course, 8 had a secondary progressive (SP) disease course, and 1 patient had a primary progressive (PP) disease course [29]. Disease duration, defined as the length of time since the patient's first symptom suggestive of MS, ranged from 2 to 22 years, with a mean of 11 years. Water content and myelin water content were measured using a 32-echo pulse sequence. Water content was estimated with reference either to the putamen water content or to contralateral brain.

Our study showed that the NAWM water content relative to putamen was, on average, 2.2±0.2% greater than that of NWM, with significant increases occurring in the posterior internal capsules (1.9%), genu (3.0%), and splenium (2.0%) of the corpus callosum, minor forceps (1.8%) and major forceps (2.6%) ($p<0.0006$) (Fig. 8). This percentage agreed with results from a different study, where the authors found a 4% increase in mean T_1 of NAWM from 13 MS patients, corresponding to an approximate 1.7% increase in water content [30, 31]. This increase in NAWM water content is further supported by our previous

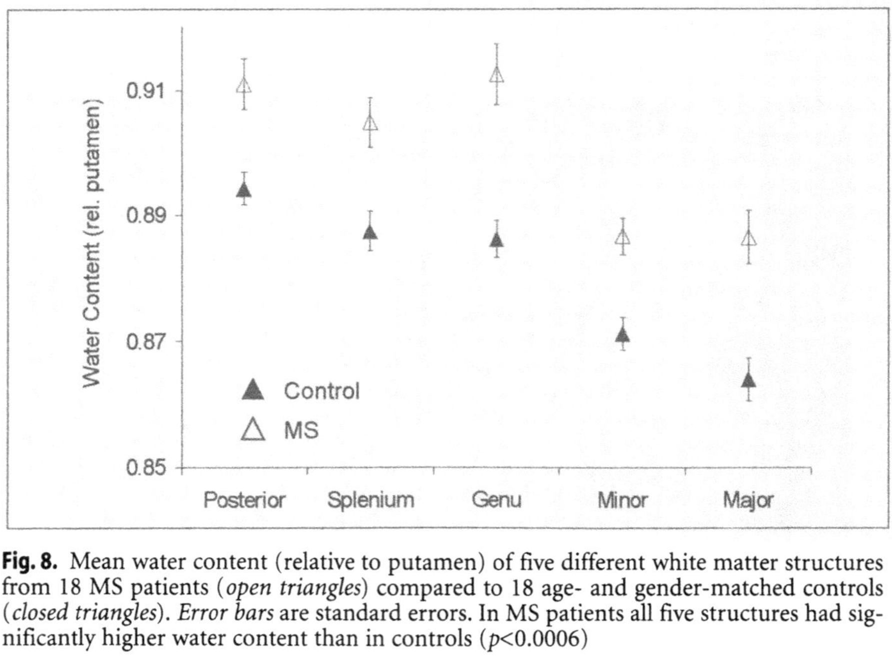

Fig. 8. Mean water content (relative to putamen) of five different white matter structures from 18 MS patients (*open triangles*) compared to 18 age- and gender-matched controls (*closed triangles*). *Error bars* are standard errors. In MS patients all five structures had significantly higher water content than in controls ($p<0.0006$)

work on MS NAWM that showed a heterogeneous and diffuse increase in the geometric mean T_2 of NAWM in MS patients [32], which may be associated with a global increase in water content. Several diffusion tensor imaging studies of MS NAWM have observed increases in apparent diffusion coefficient [33] and mean diffusivity [34, 35], thought to be related to water content. Pathology studies further support our measured increase in water content of NAWM. In a post-mortem study, Tourtellotte and Parker [36] found a mean white matter water content of 706 g H_2O/kg tissue in 10 controls and 736 g H_2O/kg tissue in 11 MS patients. Inflammation in the NAWM of patients with MS has also been observed, as well as other abnormalities such as microglial activation, increased astrocyte proliferation, and presence of myelin breakdown products [37-39].

The average MWF was 16% lower in NAWM than in NWM, with significant decreases in the major (19%) and minor forceps (26%) (p=0.003), internal capsules (14%) (p=0.01), and splenium (13%) (p=0.05) (Fig. 9). The observed decrease in myelin signal is supported by histopathological studies finding demyelination [37] as well as decreased myelin-associated glycoprotein immunostaining in white matter that appeared normal with luxol fast blue [40]. An early study suggested that, since myelin is rich in lipid and makes up the majority of all lipid found in white matter, total lipid determination could be used as a simple indicator for myelin [41]. It was found that NAWM showed a 15.5% reduction in total lipid compared to control white matter, suggesting a

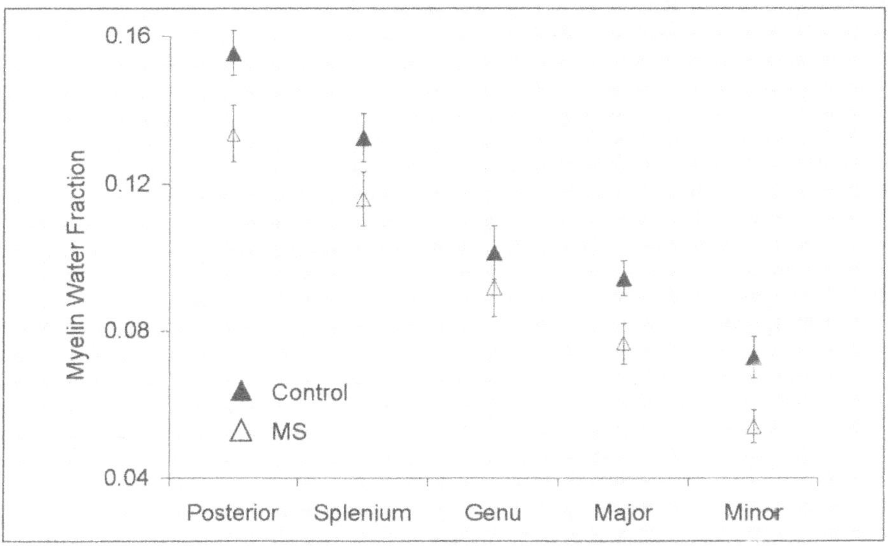

Fig. 9. Mean myelin water fraction of five different white matter structures from 18 MS patients (*open triangles*) compared to 18 age- and gender-matched controls (*closed triangles*). *Error bars* are standard errors. Four of five structures had significantly less myelin water in MS patients: splenium, posterior internal capsules, minor forceps, and major forceps (p<0.05)

similar decrease in NAWM myelin. Several other studies have examined galactolipids, including cerebrosides, which are thought to be more directly related to myelin content, and have found galactolipid decreases in NAWM of 13.5% [42] and 17% [43] compared to control white matter. The reduction in these biochemical markers of myelin has in the past been attributed to the inclusion of small plaques in the NAWM assayed [41]. MRI data, such as the present study, would suggest that such findings may be due to a more diffuse reduction of non-lesional myelin in NAWM, although the possibility of multiple small lesions beyond the resolution of current MRI techniques cannot be completely discarded. Such diffuse myelin loss could be due to concomitant loss of axons in Wallerian degeneration as reported in recent histopathological studies of NAWM [44, 45].

Model for Understanding MWF and Water Content Changes In Vivo

Our observation of both an increase in water content and decrease in MWF in the NAWM of MS patients led us to investigate further the relationship between these two results. As the MWF is a ratio of water with a T_2 less than 50 ms relative to total water content, it is conceivable that the observed decrease in MWF could be caused by an increase in total water content alone. In order to understand better the underlying physical processes we have attempted to model our findings [28] (Fig. 10). The essence of our model is the following: we separate normal white matter into two approximately equal portions, following Norton and Cammer [12] – a non-myelin fraction (which is assumed to have the properties of grey matter) and a myelin fraction, which has a lower water content. Using this model we obtain the water contents (g H_2O/g tissue) of myelin and non-myelin tissue in white matter and then calculate the average normal MWF. To simulate oedema, we added a compartment of pure water to the model and recalculated water content and MWF. To simulate myelin loss, we reduced the amount of myelin in the model, and to simulate an influx of cellular infiltrates, we increased the amount of non-myelin tissue in the model.

We use the following expressions for water content (WC), volume (V), and MWF:

$$\mathrm{WC} = \frac{\text{Total water}}{\text{Total mass}} = \frac{W_{\text{myelin}} + W_{\text{non-myelin}} + W_{\text{edema}}}{M_{\text{myelin}} + M_{\text{non-myelin}} + W_{\text{myelin}} + W_{\text{non-myelin}} + W_{\text{edema}}}$$

$$V = \frac{W_{\text{myelin}} + W_{\text{non-myelin}} + W_{\text{edema}}}{\rho_{\text{water}}} + \frac{M_{\text{myelin}}}{\rho_{\text{myelin}}} + \frac{M_{\text{non-myelin}}}{\rho_{\text{non-myelin}}}$$

$$\mathrm{MWF} = \frac{W_{\text{myelin}}}{W_{\text{myelin}} + W_{\text{non-myelin}} + W_{\text{edema}}}$$

$$= \frac{\dfrac{M_{myelin}\, WC_{myelin}}{1\text{-}WC_{myelin}}}{\dfrac{M_{myelin}\, WC_{myelin}}{1\text{-}WC_{myelin}} + \dfrac{M_{non\text{-}myelin}\, WC_{non\text{-}myelin}}{1\text{-}WC_{non\text{-}myelin}} + W_{edema}}$$

Simulation of Normal White Matter

From the literature we find NWM water content=WC_{WM}=0.72 g H_2O/g WM, $WC_{non\text{-}myelin}$=0.82 g H_2O/g non-myelin, dry fraction of white matter that is myelin=f_{myelin}=0.5, dry fraction of white matter that is non-myelin=$f_{non\text{-}myelin}$= 0.5 [12], normal brain tissue density=ρ_{brain}=1.047 g/ml [46], and density of myelin=ρ_{myelin}=1.08 g/ml [47]. We calculate the dry mass of myelin tissue, $M_{myelin}=f_{myelin}(1\ g/g\ WM-WC_{WM})$, the dry mass of non-myelin tissue, $M_{non\text{-}myelin}= f_{non\text{-}myelin}(1\ g/g\ WM-WC_{WM})$, and $V_{normal}=1/\rho_{brain}$ which is the volume of 1 g normal brain tissue. Figure 10 shows a schematic of normal white matter com-

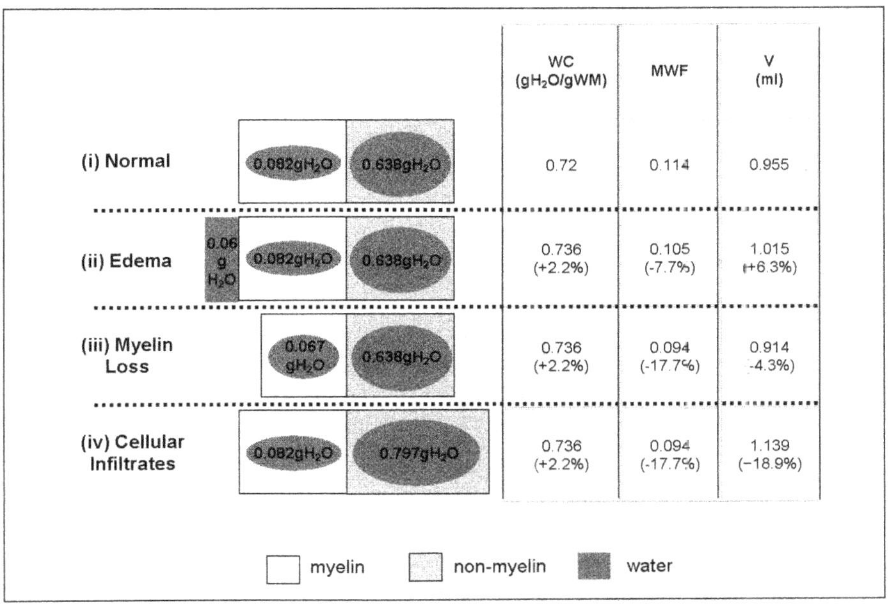

Fig. 10. A simple model of oedema, myelin loss, and inflammation in MS. Four scenarios are presented: (i) normal white matter; (ii) MS NAWM in the presence of oedema where an additional compartment of pure water is added, (iii) MS NAWM in the presence of myelin loss where the amount of myelin in white matter decreases, and (iv) MS NAWM in the presence of cellular infiltrates where the amount of non-myelin tissue increases. White, medium grey, and dark grey areas correspond to myelin, non-myelin and water respectively

ponents: water associated with non-myelin tissue $W_{non\text{-}myelin}=M_{non\text{-}myelin}(WC_{non\text{-}myelin})/(1\ g/g\ WM-WC_{non\text{-}myelin})=0.638\ g\ H_2O$, and water associated with myelin, $W_{myelin}=WC_{WM}*(1\ g\ WM)-W_{non\text{-}myelin}=0.082\ g\ H_2O$. (Note: From this we can calculate $WC_{myelin}=0.082\ g\ H_2O/(M_{myelin}+0.082\ g\ H_2O)=0.369\ g\ H_2O/g$ myelin, a quantity to be used in for the modelling of myelin loss and the influx of cellular infiltrates). For healthy white matter, we calculate a MWF of 0.114. This predicted value is in remarkable agreement with our MWF for NWM (based on average over five WM structures) of 0.111±0.004 (mean and standard error), as well as in agreement with previously published mean results of 0.113 [3].

Simulation of Oedema

To simulate oedema, we add a compartment of pure water to the model, making V_{oedema} greater than V_{normal}, and then recalculate water content and MWF as described above for normal white matter. To obtain an increase of 2.2% in NAWM water content, based on our observed results, we used a water due to oedema, $W_{oedema}=0.06$ g oedema H_2O/g WM. All other assumptions and calculations held. Consequently, for NAWM affected by oedema only, we calculate a MWF of 0.105. Therefore, modelling the observed increase in NAWM water content of 2.2% yields a reduction of only 8.8% in NAWM MWF from normal. Figure 10 shows NAWM affected by oedema. Note that oedema will result in a 6.3% swelling of NAWM (i.e. $V_{oedema}=1.063\ V_{normal}$). For the 16% reduction in NAWM MWF that was found in our study to be caused by oedema alone, one would require an approximately 4% increase in water content, resulting in a 14.5% swelling.

Simulation of Myelin Loss

To simulate myelin loss, we decrease the amount of myelin in our model, making $V_{myelin\ loss}$ less than V_{normal}. To obtain a 2.2% increase in NAWM water content, we require $M_{myelin}=0.113$ g myelin, which decreases W_{myelin}, as shown in Fig. 10. $M_{non\text{-}myelin}$ remains unchanged from the simulation of NWM=0.14 g non-myelin. Subsequently, for NAWM affected by myelin loss only, we calculate a MWF of 0.094. Note that this degree of myelin loss will result in a 4.3% shrinkage of total NAWM volume. The accompanying decrease in MWF caused by this myelin loss is 17.7%, in agreement with our observed result of 16%. To achieve a 16% decrease in NAWM MWF, our model would require $M_{myelin}= 0.115$ g myelin, resulting in a 2.0% increase in water content. The calculated 4.3% atrophy of NAWM in our myelin loss model is similar to findings from an MRI study which found a 6.4% decrease in fractional white matter volume between patients and controls [48].

Simulation of Cellular Infiltrates

To simulate an influx of cellular infiltrates, we increase the amount of non-myelin tissue in our model, causing $V_{cellular\ infiltrates}$ to be greater than V_{normal}.

To obtain a 2.2% increase in water content, again based on our observed results, we require $M_{non\text{-}myelin}$=0.174 g non-myelin, which increases $W_{non\text{-}myelin}$, as shown in Fig. 10. From this, we calculate, for NAWM with an influx of cellular infiltrates only, a MWF of 0.094, a decrease of 17.7% from normal, similar to our observed results. However, the necessary increase in volume in our model requires an 18.9% swelling of NAWM, making this scenario improbable, as such an increase would be highly unlikely from the presence of inflammatory cells alone.

Thus, the results from our NAWM model, based on average MWF and water content in NAWM compared to controls, do not support a model of global oedema or inflammation. The observed decrease in myelin water and increase in water content in NAWM best fits, however, with a model of myelin loss, such as primary demyelination or demyelination secondary to axonal loss as in Wallerian degeneration. While the combination of myelin loss and oedema or inflammation has not been modelled, we have shown that myelin loss alone is sufficient to account for our results. While oedema and inflammation may play a small role in our observed water content increase and MWF decrease, our model suggests that myelin loss is the dominant pathological process in NAWM.

Conclusions

In summary, the measurement of the complete T_2 decay curve in brain provides brain water content from summing the contributions from all T_2 components and myelin water content from the short T_2 component. Studies on fixed brain samples validate the use of the short T_2 component as a myelin marker. Comparison between T_2 decay curves from NAWM in MS and NWM indicate that NAWM has 2% higher water content and 16% lower myelin water content. This suggests that myelin loss is a dominant pathology in NAWM in MS.

References

1. Stewart WA, MacKay AL, Whittall KP et al (1993) Spin-spin relaxation in experimental allergic encephalomyelitis. Analysis of CPMG data using a non-linear least squares method and linear inverse theory. Magn Reson Med 29:767-775
2. Poon CS, Henkelman RM (1992) Practical T2 quantitation for clinical applications. J Magn Reson Imaging 2:541-553
3. Whittall KP, MacKay AL, Graeb DA et al (1996) In vivo measurement of T2 distributions and water contents in normal human brain. Magn Reson Med 37:34-43
4. Vymazal J, Brooks RA, Baumgarner C et al (1996) The relation between brain iron and NMR relaxation times: an in vitro study. Magn Reson Med 35:56-61
5. Ye FQ, Martin WR, Allen PS (1996) Estimation of brain iron in vivo by means of the interecho time dependence of image contrast. Magn Reson Med 36:153-158
6. Hallgren B, Sourander P (1958) The effect of age on the non-haemin iron in the human brain. J Neurochem 3:41-51
7. Whittall KP, MacKay AL (1989) Quantitative interpretation of NMR relaxation data. J Magn Reson 84:64-71

8. Stewart WA, MacKay AL, Whittall KP et al (1993) Spin-spin relaxation in experimental allergic encephalomyelitis. Analysis of CPMG data using a non-linear least squares method and linear inverse theory. Magn Reson Med 29:767-775
9. MacKay A, Whittall K, Adler J et al (1994) In vivo visualization of myelin water in brain by magnetic resonance. Magn Reson Med 31:673-677
10. Menon RS, Allen PS (1991) Application of continuous relaxation time distributions to the fitting of data from model systems and excised tissue. Magn Reson Med 20:214-227
11. Vasilescu V, Katona E, Simplaceanu V, Demco D (1978) Water compartments in the myelinated nerve. III. Pulsed NMR results. Experientia 34:1443-1444
12. Norton W, Cammer W (1984) Isolation and characterization of myelin. In: Morell P (ed) Myelin, 2nd edn. Plenum Press, New York, pp 147-195
13. Wolff SD, Balaban R (1989) Magnetization transfer contrast (MTC) and tissue water proton relaxation in vivo. Magn Reson Med 10:135-144
14. Stanisz GJ, Kecojevic A, Bronskill MJ, Henkelman RM (1999) Characterizing white matter with magnetization transfer and T(2). Magn Reson Med 42:1128-1136
15. Dousset V, Brochet B, Vital A et al (1995) Lysolecithin-induced demyelination in primates: preliminary in vivo study with MR and magnetization transfer. AJNR Am J Neuroradiol 16:225-231
16. Gareau PJ, Rutt BK, Bowen CV et al (1999) In vivo measurements of multi-component T2 relaxation behaviour in guinea pig brain. Magn Reson Imaging 17:1319-1325
17. Gareau PJ, Rutt BK, Karlik SJ, Mitchell JR (2000) Magnetization transfer and multicomponent T2 relaxation measurements with histopathologic correlation in an experimental model of MS. J Magn Reson Imaging 11:586-595
18. Laule C, Vavasour IM, Paty D et al (2002) Correlation between magnetization transfer ratio and myelin water content in normal white matter and MS lesions. [Abstract] Proc Int Soc Magn Reson Med 10:182
19. Vavasour IM, Whittall KP, MacKay AL et al (1998) A comparison between magnetization transfer ratios and myelin water percentages in normals and multiple sclerosis patients. Magn Reson Med 40:763-768
20. Moseley ME, Cohen Y, Kucharczyk J et al (1990) Diffusion-weighted MR imaging of anisotropic water diffusion in cat central nervous system. Radiology 176:439-445
21. Chenevert TL, Brunberg JA, Pipe JG (1990) Anisotropic diffusion in human white matter: demonstration with MR techniques in vivo. Radiology 177:401-405
22. Moseley ME, Kucharczyk J, Asgari HS, Norman D (1991) Anisotropy in diffusion-weighted MRI. Magn Reson Med 19:321-326
23. Maedler B, Whittall KP, MacKay AL (2002) Correlation of multicomponent T2-relaxation data with diffusion tensor anisotropy measures in human brain. [Abstract] Proc Int Soc Magn Reson Med 10:1188
24. Webb S, Munro CA, Midha R, Stanisz GJ (2003) Is multicomponent T2 a good measure of myelin content in peripheral nerve? Magn Reson Med 49:638-645
25. Araujo C, MacKay AL, Whittall KP et al (1993) A diffusion model for spin-spin relaxation of compartmentalized water in wood. J Magn Reson 101:248-261
26. Moore GR, Leung E, MacKay AL et al (2000) A pathology-MRI study of the short-T2 component in formalin-fixed multiple sclerosis brain. Neurology 55:1506-1510
27. Laule C, Leung E, Li DKB et al (2003) Myelin water imaging in multiple sclerosis: quantitative correlations with histopathology. Mult Scler 9(Suppl 1):S12
28. Laule C, Vavasour IM, Moore GRW et al (2004) Water content and myelin water fraction in multiple sclerosis: a T2 relaxation study. J Neurol 251:284-293
29. Lublin FD, Reingold SC (1996) Defining the clinical course of multiple sclerosis: results of an international survey. National Multiple Sclerosis Society (USA) Advisory Committee on Clinical Trials of New Agents in Multiple Sclerosis. Neurology 46:907-911

30. Rooney W, Springer C, Telang F et al (2002) Comparison of brain 4T T1 histograms between multiple sclerosis and control subjects. Mult Scler 8:80
31. Fatouros PP, Marmarou A (1999) Use of magnetic resonance imaging for in vivo measurements of water content in human brain: method and normal values. J Neurosurg 90:109-115
32. Whittall KP, MacKay AL, Li DK et al (2002) Normal-appearing white matter in multiple sclerosis has heterogeneous, diffusely prolonged T(2). Magn Reson Med 47:403-408
33. Werring DJ, Clark CA, Droogan AG et al (2001) Water diffusion is elevated in widespread regions of normal-appearing white matter in multiple sclerosis and correlates with diffusion in focal lesions. Mult Scler 7:83-89
34. Bammer R, Augustin M, Strasser-Fuchs S et al (2000) Magnetic resonance diffusion tensor imaging for characterizing diffuse and focal white matter abnormalities in multiple sclerosis. Magn Reson Med 44:583-591
35. Filippi M, Iannucci G, Cercignani M et al (2000) A quantitative study of water diffusion in multiple sclerosis lesions and normal-appearing white matter using echo-planar imaging. Arch Neurol 57:1017-1021
36. Tourtellotte W, Parker J (1968) Some spaces and barriers in postmortem multiple sclerosis. Prog Brain Res 29:493-525
37. Allen IV, Glover G, Anderson R (1981) Abnormalities in the macroscopically normal white matter in cases of mild or spinal multiple sclerosis (MS). Acta Neuropathol 7(Suppl):176-178
38. Allen IV, McKeown SR (1979) A histological, histochemical and biochemical study of the macroscopically normal white matter in multiple sclerosis. J Neurol Sci 41:81-91
39. Allen IV, McQuaid S, Mirakhur M, Nevin G (2001) Pathological abnormalities in the normal-appearing white matter in multiple sclerosis. Neurol Sci 22:141-144
40. Itoyama Y, Sternberger NH, Webster HD et al (1980) Immunocytochemical observations on the distribution of myelin-associated glycoprotein and myelin basic protein in multiple sclerosis lesions. Ann Neurol 7:167-177
41. Suzuki K, Kamoshita S, Eto Y et al (1973) Myelin in multiple sclerosis. Composition of myelin from normal-appearing white matter. Arch Neurol 28:293-297
42. Alling C, Vanier MT, Svennerholm L (1971) Lipid alterations in apparently normal white matter in multiple sclerosis. Brain Res 35:325-336
43. Fewster ME, Hirono H, Mead JF (1976) Lipid composition of myelin in multiple sclerosis. J Neurol 213:119-131
44. Evangelou N, Esiri MM, Smith S et al (2000) Quantitative pathological evidence for axonal loss in normal appearing white matter in multiple sclerosis. Ann Neurol 47:391-395
45. Evangelou N, Konz D, Esiri MM et al (2000) Regional axonal loss in the corpus callosum correlates with cerebral white matter lesion volume and distribution in multiple sclerosis. Brain 123:1845-1849
46. Brooks RA, Di Chiro G, Keller MR (1980) Explanation of cerebral white-grey contrast in computed tomography. J Comput Assist Tomogr 4:489-491
47. Morell P, Quarles RH, Norton W (1989) Formation, structure, and biochemistry of myelin. In: Siegel J (ed) Basic neurochemistry: molecular, cellular, and medical aspects, 4th edn. Raven Press, New York, pp 109-136
48. Ge Y, Grossman RI, Udupa JK et al (2001) Brain atrophy in relapsing-remitting multiple sclerosis: fractional volumetric analysis of grey matter and white matter. Radiology 220:606-610

Chapter 6

Rapid, Whole-Brain T_1 Relaxation Time Measurements for the Quantitative Definition of Pathological Changes in Multiple Sclerosis

A.M. Parry, S. Clare, P.M. Matthews

Introduction

Multiple sclerosis (MS) is a disabling neurological condition characterized clinically by episodes of acute neurological dysfunction and/or progressive irreversible disability.

Although MS is characterized pathologically by the presence of multifocal white matter lesions (containing areas of inflammation, demyelination, gliosis, and axonal loss), axonal loss also occurs extensively outside of focal lesions throughout the normal-appearing white matter (NAWM) of the brain [1] and spinal cord [2, 3]. Further pathological studies also have demonstrated that focal lesions [4, 5] and neuronal injury occur in the cortical [6] and deep grey matter [7]. These pathological changes in the NAWM and grey matter may be a principal determinant of physical and cognitive disability from MS.

Role of MRI in MS

The ability of magnetic resonance imaging (MRI) non-invasively to visualize pathological change in vivo has had a profound impact on the clinical management of patients with MS and on the understanding of the disease and its treatment. In addition to substantially contributing to the diagnosis of MS and providing some limited information regarding prognosis [8], MRI and related techniques also have been able to shed considerable light on the natural history of the pathology of MS relevant to understanding treatment effects [9]. However, critical questions concerning the development of pathological change from MS still remain. The principal mechanisms driving clinically relevant axonal loss in the NAWM and grey matter and the pathological basis for the observed clinical heterogeneity in MS patients are not fully understood. A greater understanding of these pathological processes is likely to contribute to the development of effective new treatment strategies.

To successfully address these questions, new MRI techniques ideally should have good spatial resolution (to define changes in anatomically distinguishable compartments, e.g., both in focal lesions and in the NAWM) and allow a "whole-brain" approach within a clinically acceptable scan time. The measurement of pathological changes should also be both quantitative and objective. Finally, there is a need for measures that have clinical relevance, demonstrated by a close relationship between measures of pathological change and progression of disability.

T_1-Based Hypointensity and MS

T1 Hypointensity ("Black Holes"): An MRI Surrogate Marker of Clinically Relevant Pathological Change in Focal Lesions

Correlative pathological studies have demonstrated that hypointensity on T_1-weighted MRI is associated with matrix destruction and axonal loss [10, 11], a putative cause of irreversible neurological deficits in MS [12]. The clinical relevance of T_1-hypointense lesions as a surrogate marker of pathological change has been established by observations which have shown both a significant cross-sectional correlation between T_1 lesion load (non-enhancing T_1 hypointensity volume measured on gadolinium-enhanced T_1-weighted images) and disability in MS patients [13, 14], and longitudinal observations that have shown that the accumulation of T1 lesion volume over time strongly correlates with changes in disability for patients with secondary progressive MS [14].

Limitations of the Measurement of T_1-Hypointense Lesion Load

However, whilst providing a clinically relevant index of disease burden from MS, the measurement of focal T_1-hypointense lesion volume has several limitations. Reports to date have relied on the manual outlining of hypointense lesions "by eye" on the T_1-weighted MRI scan, an approach with two major weaknesses. First, the sequence parameters used (e.g., the TR) and other instrument factors (e.g., radiofrequency coil inhomogeneities) to acquire the T_1-weighted image will determine the relative contrast between the lesions and surrounding brain and thus influence the identification of lesions substantially. Therefore, images of the same brain acquired on different instruments may lead to some difference in lesion definition. In addition, as multiple factors interact in the identification of the boundaries of hypointense lesions (e.g. the luminance of the image), there can be significant variance difference in segmentation [15].

A second important limitation of subjective manual methods for identifying T_1 hypointensity is that any less dramatic T_1-contrast changes in the NAWM or grey matter which may contribute to physical or cognitive disability cannot be defined easily.

T_1 Relaxometry: An Alternative Approach for Detecting Changes Contributing Towards T_1 Hypointensity

The direct measurement of T_1 relaxation times (T_1) allows a potentially more sensitive, specific, and objective approach for detecting changes contributing to hypointensity on the T_1-weighted image. The T_1 value increases with the field strength used for the scan acquisition but is otherwise independent of acquisition parameters if measured appropriately [16-19]. The use of a voxel-by-voxel acquisition method with good spatial resolution also allows the quantitative evaluation of the severity of T_1 changes in different tissue compartments, e.g. both in lesions and in the NAWM (as defined by conventional imaging).

Quantifying T_1 Relaxation Time

To quantify T_1 it is necessary to take a series of separate MRI scans. A semiquantitative measure can be made from two scans, but to measure T_1 more accurately a larger number is required. Each scan can take many minutes to acquire, and this meant that some of the early work measuring T_1 was restricted to just a few slices of the brain [20-21]. However, more recent technological developments have meant that it is now possible to get whole-brain, quantitative maps of T_1 in several minutes.

The conventional method for quantification of T_1 is to use an inversion recovery pulse sequence. This method is uses a 180° inversion pulse prior to imaging. Figure 1 shows a plot of the magnetization following an inversion pulse. The *y* axis represents the amount of signal that would be detected in an image acquired at that particular time. Therefore, an image collected at A would have a very low signal intensity whereas an image acquired at B would have a much higher intensity. By collecting images at a range of times following the inversion pulse it is

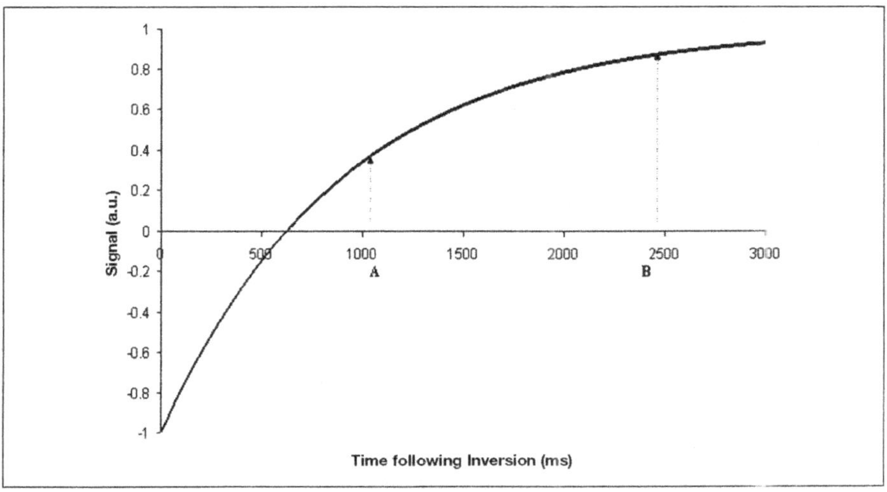

Fig. 1. Plot of the signal recovery following an inversion radiofrequency pulse. Images acquired at an inversion time *A* will have a different signal intensity than those acquired at time *B*. *a.u.*, arbitrary units

possible to fit an exponential curve to the values and determine the rate time constant, T_1. An important thing to note from this figure is the time scale involved. For the full recovery of signal from brain tissue it is necessary to wait at least 15 s between measurements. Since conventionally one measurement is required for each line in the image, and several points on the recovery curve need to be sampled for accurate quantification, the mapping of T_1 values in the brain can take up to an hour and only cover a limited number of slices.

Due to the time involved, it has been more common to use semi-quantitative measures of T_1, (made from just two time points). More recently, however, there have been several methods that attempt to considerably reduce the scan time and allow whole-brain, fully quantitative T1 mapping in several minutes. This has been achieved by using the rapid imaging technique of echo planar imaging (EPI). This method acquires an image of single slice of the brain in under 100 ms. This is typically at low resolution and suffers from image distortion, particularly in the frontal and temporal lobes. However, optimization of the technique makes it possible to use EPI to image the whole brain at a resolution of 2×2×2 mm^3 with minimal distortion.

Whilst using EPI for imaging can significantly reduce the time taken to acquire a T_1 map, further time savings can also be made by adapting the inversion recovery method. A considerable increase in the speed of T1 mapping can be achieved by implementing the Look-Locker method [22]. This method uses many low flip angle acquisitions to inspect a single recovery curve following an inversion pulse, so reducing the need for long delays between several inversions. There are some penalties with this approach, however, notably in the sensitivity of the result to the flip angle used for the excitation pulses. A combination of EPI and the Look-Locker approach (LL-EPI) probably represents the fastest T_1 mapping sequence that can be achieved, with a T1 recovery curve from a single slice being acquired in 3 s [23].

As an alternative, it is possible to reduce the long delays inherent in the inversion recovery method. Since it is desirable to image each slice at a range of inversion pulses, this method uses a "non-selective" inversion pulse that inverts the signal in all slices and then sequentially acquires each slice. Thus, every slice is acquired at a different delay following the inversion pulse. By repeating this, but changing the slice order, it is possible to build up data from every slice in the brain at a full range of inversion times [24]. This builds up enough data for a fully quantitative T_1 map of the whole brain (60×2-mm-thick slices) in just 3 s [25].

To obtain a T_1 value it is necessary to fit the acquired data from each pixel in the image and at each inversion time to an exponential recovery curve. One problem with this is that the image data is inherently "rectified". In Fig. 1 the magnetization prior to 600 ms is negative (inverted), but the signal detected will be positive (i.e. the modulus of the result). This can cause problems in fitting the data, although there are various solutions for finding accurate and reliable fits to the data in the presence of noise [25, 26]. Once a T_1 value has been fit for every pixel in the image, the data can be displayed as an image (Fig. 2). However, since

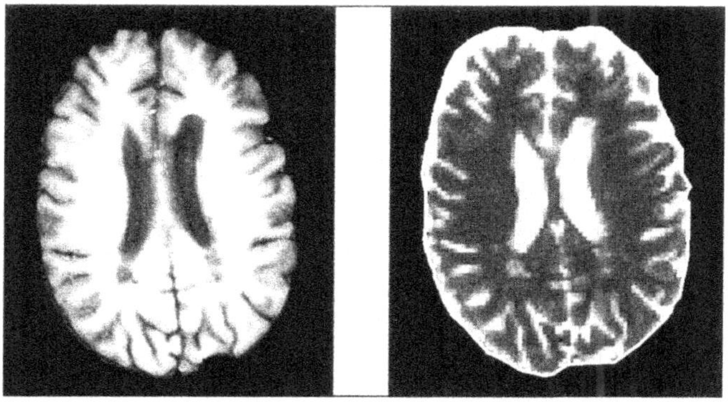

Fig. 2. Corresponding slices from a T_1-weighted image (*left*) and a T_1 relaxation time map (*right*) from a patient with secondary progressive multiple sclerosis [25]

these values are quantitative, a more useful comparison is to compare the values directly. This can be done by taking the mean of a region of interest (ROI), e.g. in the NAWM, or alternatively by representing the range of T_1 values contained within a defined area as a histogram. The benefit of using a histogram is that it is possible to detect more subtle "shoulders" in the data. This is potentially a more sensitive measure than the mean if only a proportion of values within the ROI demonstrate a change in T_1. The peak height of the histogram (percentage of image pixels contained within a defined area at the modal value) also can be calculated to provide an index of tissue dispersion.

Clinical Applications of T_1 Relaxometry in MS

T_1 Relaxometry Is Sensitive to Pathological Changes in Both White Matter Lesions and the NAWM

Several studies using a histogram-based analysis approach have shown that T_1 relaxometry is sensitive to pathological changes in the cerebral white matter of patients with MS when compared to controls [27-30] and that these changes can be detected even early on in the disease course [28].

A recent study showed that total cerebral white matter T_1 values measured at 3 T in MS patients were shifted significantly towards higher T_1 values compared to control subjects (mean T_1 value: patients, 964 ms, SD 66; controls 891 ms, SD 23, $p<0.01$) [27]. The spread of the patient group histogram towards higher T_1 values also led to a significant reduction in the peak height of the MS patient histogram (Fig. 3). Similar increases in cervical cord T_1 values in MS patients relative to controls have been observed [29]. Although neither of these studies [27, 29] were powered to test whether T_1 measurements can differentiate between clinical subgroups of MS, it is of interest that the patients with secondary progressive multiple sclerosis (SPMS) had a trend towards higher T_1 values than the patients with relapsing-remitting multiple sclerosis (RRMS) (Fig. 3), consistent

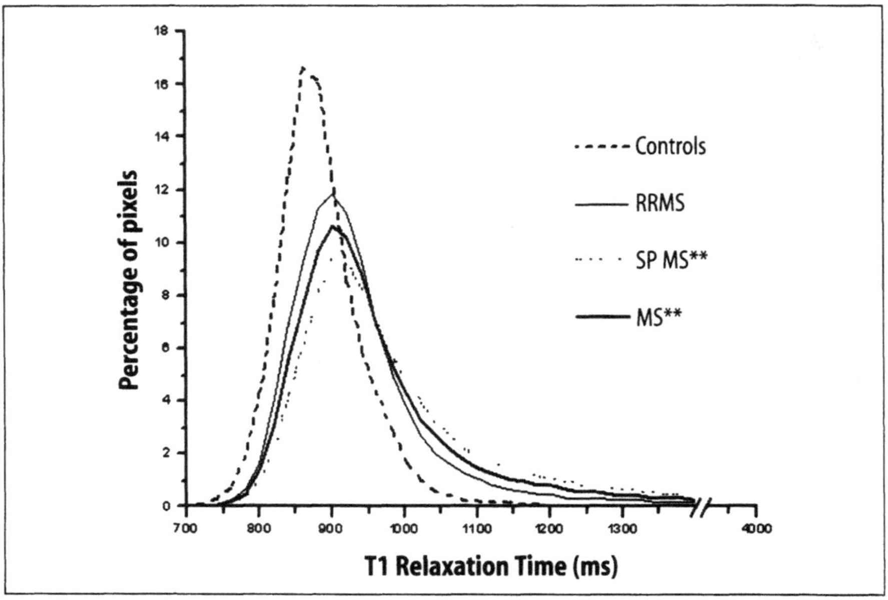

Fig. 3. Average white matter T_1 relaxation histograms from the control, relapsing-remitting patients (RRMS), secondary progressive patients (SPMS), and combined patient group (MS). ** Significant difference between patients and controls ($p<0.05$) [27]

with the hypothesis that there is greater generalized tissue injury in patients with SPMS than in those with RRMS [31-33].

T_1 relaxometry also is sensitive to the diffuse pathological changes in the NAWM that constitute the "invisible" lesion load. Because the NAWM is so much larger than the lesion volume (e.g. typical lesion volumes of 20 cm^3 in a white matter volume of 500 cm^3), the burden of disease from this diffuse load is potentially high. In fact, T_1 histograms in the cerebral NAWM show evidence for a substantial volume of white matter with a significantly prolonged T_1 compared to controls [27]. This is consistent with previous pathological studies which demonstrated that axonal loss occurs throughout both the cerebral [1] and spinal cord NAWM [2, 3].

These data using histogram-based analyses (which aim to sample large representative tissue volumes) extend previous studies (performed using a region of interest approach) which have shown that T_1 prolongation occurs in both macroscopic lesions and in the NAWM.

T_1 Relaxometry Is Sensitive to Clinically Relevant Pathological Change

In addition to detecting and quantifying pathological change from MS, useful "surrogate" MRI modalities should also be sensitive to pathological change that is relevant clinically.

A relationship between higher T_1 values in both the cerebral white matter [27] and cervical cord [29] and greater disability (Expanded Disability Status Scale, EDSS) has been observed (e.g. with r>0.55, p≤0.01 for cortical white matter). Increases in T_1 values in the NAWM of patients presenting with clinically isolated syndromes also have been shown to correlate with cognitive disability [34].

Relatively high-resolution T_1 relaxometry also has allowed the severity of disease burden in region-specific areas to be correlated with clinically relevant disability. Using diffusion tensor imaging to define the pyramidal tracts, Vaithianathar et al. demonstrated that there was a significant relationship between white matter T_1 values and the pyramidal functional score of the EDSS [30]. These data are consistent with previous studies of T_1 signal change based on manual segmentation which have shown that greater "black hole" volume is associated with increased disability [13, 14]. These two observations differ, however, in that T_1 relaxometry methods can allow the substantial contribution of what conventional imaging would define as NAWM to tissue T_1 changes to be considered. Quantitative measurements from large volumes of white matter containing a high percentage of NAWM may therefore provide similar information to that from "black hole" volumes with the advantage that T_1 values are stable between centres with analysis that is easily automated for acquisition efficiency and objectivity.

The relatively poor relationship between pathologically heterogeneous T_2 lesion volume and disability [35] suggests that it is the qualitative nature and severity of the pathological change found in focal lesions rather than absolute lesion load that partly determines clinical disability. In keeping with this hypothesis, a significant correlation has been observed between the mean T_1 of hypointense lesions and the EDSS, but no relationship between the mean T_1 in T_2-weighted lesions and EDSS [27]. Similarly, whilst T_1 values in the pyramidal tract of patients with MS were correlated with pyramidal tract functional system EDSS scores, no such relationship existed between T_1 lesion volume in the pyramidal tract region and disability [30].

T_1 Relaxometry Provides Insights into Possible Mechanisms Driving Pathological Change in the NAWM

The direct measurement of T_1 values allows an objective assessment of the severity of T_1 changes in the focal lesions and in the NAWM and their relationship to each other. Pathological studies have demonstrated that axonal loss is not confined to focal lesions, but occurs extensively throughout the NAWM in the brain [1, 36, 37] and spinal cord [2, 3] and probably is a critical determinant of progressive irreversible disability [38, 39]. Understanding how axonal injury in the NAWM occurs is therefore critical to the development of disease-modifying treatments.

The observations that axonal injury or transaction in MS lesions co-localizes with acute inflammatory activity [36, 37] suggests that ongoing focal inflamma-

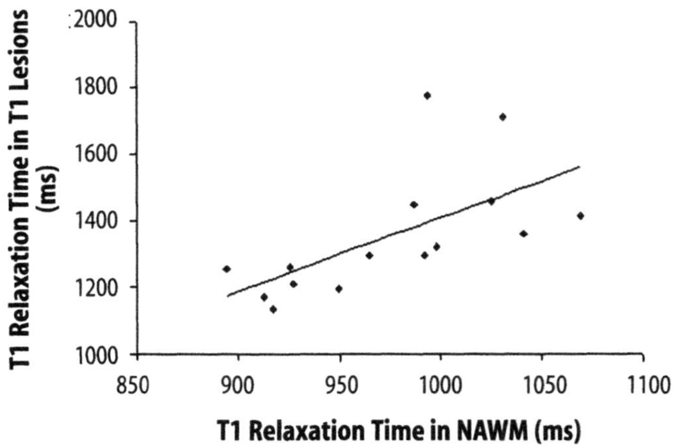

Fig. 4. Correlation between mean T_1 relaxation time in the normal-appearing white matter (NAWM) and mean T_1 relaxation time in the hypointense lesions seen on the T_1-weighted image (r=0.80, p<0.001) [27]

tion and demyelination may be a critical determinant of axonal pathology. The potential importance of lesions as a focal determinant of axonal injury is further supported by evidence that suggests that axonal loss in the NAWM is correlated with regional lesion load [42]. This favours the hypothesis that axonal injury occurs as a direct "downstream" consequence of focal inflammation, as opposed to being caused by a diffuse axonopathy. Axonal injury may not solely depend on the presence of acute inflammation, however. MRI studies of patients with primary progressive MS have shown that widespread tissue damage can occur despite the relative paucity of focal inflammatory lesions [40, 41], suggesting that axonal injury may not be solely dependent on the presence of acute inflammation.

To test the hypothesis that pathological change in the NAWM occurs as a consequence of focal lesions (as opposed to occurring as a second independent process), T_1 values were measured directly both in the NAWM and in focal hypointense lesions. A significant correlation between the mean T_1 value in the NAWM and the mean T_1 in the hypointense lesions (Fig. 4) was observed, suggesting that T_1-hypointense pathological changes in the NAWM may arise directly as a consequence of focal pathological change in lesions [27].

T_1 Relaxometry Is Sensitive to Pathological Change in the Grey Matter

Pathological change in the grey matter of patients with MS [4-7] may be an important determinant of cognitive impairment in MS. Therefore to avoid underestimating the true disease burden in an individual, MRI techniques that aim to quantify clinically relevant pathological change from MS should also be sensitive to pathological changes in the grey matter.

To test whether T_1 relaxometry is sensitive to the detection of pathological change in the grey matter, mean T_1 values in the thalamus in patients with RRMS and SPMS and in controls have been compared. Whilst there was no significant difference in the mean T_1 values in the thalamus between the patient group and the control group, the mean thalamic T_1 value in the sub-group of patients with SPMS was significantly higher than either the control group or the RRMS sub-group [27]. This difference in T_1 values may reflect a relative loss of neurite density, similar to that associated with T_1 changes in the white matter [10, 11]. These results must be interpreted with some caution, however, as grey matter is heterogeneous in structure (and therefore potential susceptibility to injury) and regions of the thalamus contain relatively high proportions of myelin [43].

T_1 Relaxometry Is Sensitive to the Progression of Disease

To determine the potential sensitivity of T_1 mapping for the detection of ongoing pathological change in the white matter and in the cortical grey matter, patients who had participated in a previous study [27] were re-examined after a median time of 19.5 months to determine whether significant changes in T_1 relaxation time could be observed in white matter or cortical grey matter over this time period [44]. A significant reduction in the total (lesions and NAWM) cerebral white matter histogram peak height (13%) between the baseline and the follow-up examination was observed. Despite these changes in the whole white matter T_1 histogram, there was no significant change in the volume of white matter with the most abnormal T_1 values (greater than 3 standard deviations above the mean control white matter T_1 value) over time. The change in the total white matter histogram over time, however, could be accounted for by a significant reduction (8%) in the NAWM histogram peak height with time. This significant reduction in peak height in the absence of any significant change in histogram median or modal value suggests that pathological change in the NAWM does not occur uniformly, consistent with a microscopic multi-focal process not visible with conventional MRI approaches.

The observed changes in T_1 values in the NAWM in the absence of a change in the volume of T_1 hypointensity may suggest that ongoing damage in the NAWM is *not* driven by the accumulation of focal lesions. Previous work, for example, has demonstrated that changes in the NAWM may precede the development of lesions [45-47]. However, it also is possible that the differences between NAWM and lesional changes merely reflect increased sensitivity of the former if degeneration of axons leading into or out of focal lesions "amplifies" these effects all along the affected tracts. A more sensitive measure of focal disease activity in MS patients may also be afforded by MRI techniques that measure lesion volume turnover rather than net lesion load. Studies that have evaluated the contribution to net changes in lesion volume from both new and evolving lesions have demonstrated a greater degree of lesion activity than previously reported than when just net changes in lesion load are measured [48].

In contrast to the observed changes in T_1 values with time in the white matter, the study by Parry et al. [44] demonstrated that mean and median T_1 values in the cortical grey matter of MS patients significantly decreased (6%) with time. There was also a significant increase (9%) in the histogram peak height over time. The greatest changes in T_1 values occurred in patients with longer disease duration. The pathological substrate for this observed decrease in grey matter T_1 values is uncertain, but may be related to non-specific increased iron deposition with neurodegeneration [49], analogous to the hypotheses used to explain the reductions in T_2 relaxation time reported in MS patients in both the cortex [50] and the basal ganglia [51-53].

Differences in the dynamic pattern of T_1 changes between white matter and grey matter may reflect differences in the nature of the pathological changes from MS in these tissues. A recent pathological study suggested that there may be inflammatory differences in the pathology between cortical grey and white matter lesions in MS. Compared with white matter lesions, cortical lesions contained fewer inflammatory cells and less perivascular "cuffing" [6].

In the follow-up study of T_1 changes in the white and grey matter [44], there was no relationship between the change in disability as measured by the EDSS score and change in any of the white or grey matter T_1 histogram parameters. However, this study was not powered to detect such a relationship, and the nonlinearity of the EDSS may make it poorly suited for correlation with the imaging measures of pathology. The study [54], however, clearly demonstrates that the measurement of T_1 relaxation time is sensitive to the progression of pathological change from MS occurring over a relatively short time period. If these changes are assumed (for convenience of estimation) to be linear, then we expect that significant changes would be detected in a patient group of this size over an interval as short as 6 months.

The early detection of T_1 abnormalities in both the grey and white matter [28] and the sensitivity of T_1 relaxometry to change over time may therefore provide a sensitive, quantitative index of clinically relevant pathological change from MS. This measure would be practical to apply in clinical trials: the protocol used in the studies by Parry et al. [27, 44] can be run in 3 min and analysis potentially relies largely on highly automated and therefore objective routines [49].

Potential Problems in the Interpretation of T_1 Relaxometry Changes

The work that we have described from our own laboratory has been performed at 3 T. T_1 relaxation time values increase with field strength [16, 18]. Absolute differences in T_1 values between patient populations and controls therefore may be different at 3 T to T_1 value differences detected at the more conventional field strength of 1.5 T. However, other T_1 relaxometry studies performed at 1.5 T have shown that similar qualitative differences in T_1 values between population groups also can be detected at this more conventional field strength [29, 30].

A second limitation of some of the T_1 studies discussed above [27, 29, 30] is that gadolinium-DTPA was not used to exclude regions of acute inflammation contributing to T_1 changes from the analysis. T_1 increases also are shown in regions of increased water content not associated with local tissue destruction. This is particularly true of the diffuse changes [54, 55]. This may have decreased the correlation between T_1 values and clinical measures of irreversible disability. However, this approach is less invasive and potentially more cost effective.

A more recent pathological study demonstrated that whilst axonal density in focal lesions is generally reduced in lesions that are more T_1-hypointense (measured descriptively and also as a ratio of contrast to the NAWM), it is not necessarily the case that there is a simple correlation between axonal density and T_1 across the full range of values. It also was also shown that a "mildly T_1-hypointense" focal lesion could have a normal axonal density. However, in this study, axonal density in lesions was quantified by visual comparison to the axonal density in the NAWM [11]. Since significant axon loss can occur in the NAWM [1], this study may have been insensitive to more subtle changes in axonal density in the focal lesions. Reassuringly, the axonal density in "very T_1-hypointense" lesions in this correlative pathological study [11] was never normal. Since T_1 relaxometry methods are quantitative, a "thresholding" approach to quantify areas of more severe T_1-hypointense change (which are more likely to be associated with irreversible axonal loss) may be easily employed.

Future Directions: Understanding the Clinical Heterogeneity of MS Disease Severity

Patients with SPMS have a higher T_1 lesion volume/T_2 lesion volume ratio than do patients with RRMS [56], consistent with the notion of greater burden of irreversible axonal loss in patients with SPMS [31-33]. However, even within these patient sub-populations, there exists considerable clinical heterogeneity in the severity of the disease course. This may be due to the severity of any initial pathological changes, e.g. the prevalence of acute axonal injury within new focal lesions, or to varying degrees of subsequent reparative processes, e.g. remyelination.

The increase in T_1-hypointense lesions over time has been shown to be better predicted by baseline T_1-hypointense lesion volume rather than the baseline level of gadolinium enhancing activity. This may suggests that there is a sub-population of MS patients who have a predisposition to developing destructive lesions [57].

In support of this hypothesis, a recent pathological study has suggested that there may be a relatively homogeneous pattern of lesion activity within (rather than between) patients with MS [58]. Cross-sectional pathological studies, however, are unable to comment on the persistence of lesion clinical homogeneity within a patient over time. In contrast, the quantitative approach of T_1 mapping may allow the MRI characteristics of focal lesions within an individual to be re-examined over long time periods. This may provide insight into the stability of lesion type over time and identify whether subtle changes in lesion characteristics correlate with the clinical course of the disease (e.g. the transition from RRMS to SPMS).

Clinical heterogeneity may also be partly determined by the spatial characteristics of pathological change from MS, e.g. the accumulation of T_1 changes in the pyramidal tract may be a more important determinant of ambulation status than T_1 changes in the corpus callosum [30]. The quantitative whole-brain approach of T_1 mapping may therefore allow the spatial mapping of clinically relevant pathological change from MS to be determined more precisely.

The combined approach of longitudinal T_1 mapping and diffusion-weighted tractography (to define anatomically connected brain areas) in patients presenting with clinically isolated syndromes may also provide important insight into the mechanisms driving pathological change in the NAWM. Further multimodal MRI approaches (e.g. the combination of MTR and T_1 mapping) may also provide complementary information in the quantification and understanding of pathological change from MS [5-7, 42].

Acknowledgements. The authors gratefully acknowledge the support of the Medical Research Council (UK), the MS Society of Great Britain and Northern Ireland, and the Amyotrophic Lateral Sclerosis Association of America.

References

1. Evangelou N, Esiri MM, Smith S et al (2000) Quantitative pathological evidence for axonal loss in normal appearing white matter in multiple sclerosis. Ann Neurol 47:391-395
2. Lovas G, Szilagyi N, Majtenyi K et al (2000) Axonal changes in chronic demyelinated cervical spinal cord plaques. Brain 123:308-317
3. Ganter P, Prince C, Esiri MM (1999) Spinal cord axonal loss in multiple sclerosis: a post-mortem study. Neuropathol Appl Neurobiol 25:459-467
4. Brownell B, Hughes JT (1962) The distribution of plaques in the cerebrum in multiple sclerosis. J Neurol Neurosurg Psychiatry 25:315-320
5. Kidd D, Barkhof F, McConnell R et al (1999) Cortical lesions in multiple sclerosis. Brain 122 (Pt 1):17-26
6. Peterson JW, Bö L, Mork S et al (2001) Transected neurites, apoptotic neurons, and reduced inflammation in cortical multiple sclerosis lesions. Ann Neurol 50:389-400
7. Cifelli A, Arridge M, Jezzard P et al (2002) Thalamic neurodegeneration in multiple sclerosis. Ann Neurol 52:650-653
8. Brex PA, Ciccarelli O, O'Riordan JI et al (2002) A longitudinal study of abnormalities on MRI and disability from multiple sclerosis. N Engl J Med 346:158-164
9. Miller DH (1998) Multiple sclerosis: use of MRI in evaluating new therapies. Semin Neurol 18:317-325
10. van Walderveen MA, Kamphorst W, Scheltens P et al (1998) Histopathologic correlate of hypointense lesions on T1-weighted spin-echo MRI in multiple sclerosis. Neurology 50:1282-1288
11. van Waesberghe JH, Kamphorst W, De Groot CJ et al (1999) Axonal loss in multiple sclerosis lesions: magnetic resonance imaging insights into substrates of disability. Ann Neurol 46:747-754

12. Matthews PM, De Stefano N, Narayanan S et al (1998) Putting MRS studies in context: axonal damage and disability in MS. Semin Neurol 51:327-336
13. van Walderveen MA, Barkhof F, Hommes OR et al (1995) Correlating MRI and clinical disease activity in multiple sclerosis: relevance of hypointense lesions on short-TR/short-TE (T1-weighted) spin-echo images. Neurology 45:1684-1690
14. Truyen L, van Waesberghe JH, van Walderveen MA et al (1996) Accumulation of hypointense lesions ("black holes") on T1 spin-echo MRI correlates with disease progression in multiple sclerosis. Neurology 47:1469-1476
15. Molyneux PD, Brex PA, Fogg C et al (2000) The precision of T1 hypointense lesion volume quantification in multiple sclerosis treatment trials: a multicenter study. Mult Scler 6:237-240
16. Kim SG, Hu X, Ugurbil K (1994) Accurate T1 determination from inversion recovery images: application to human brain at 4 Tesla. Magn Reson Med 31:445-449
17. Breger RK, Wehrli FW, Charles HC (1986) Reproducibility of relaxation and spin-density parameters in phantoms and the human brain measured by MR imaging at 1.5 T. Magn Reson Med 3:649-662
18. Jezzard P, Duewell S, Balaban RS (1996) MR relaxation times in human brain: measurement at 4 T. Radiology 199:773-779
19. Wansapura JP, Holland SK, Dunn RS, Ball WS Jr (1999) NMR relaxation times in the human brain at 3.0 tesla, J Magn Reson Imaging 9:531-538
20. Lacomis D, Osbakken M, Gross G (1986) Spin-lattice relaxation (T1) times of cerebral white matter in multiple sclerosis. Magn Reson Med 3:194-202
21. Larsson HB, Frederiksen J, Petersen J et al (1989) Assessment of demyelination, edema, and gliosis by in vivo determination of T1 and T2 in the brain of patients with acute attack of multiple sclerosis. Magn Reson Med 11:337-348
22. Crawley AP, Henkelman RM (1988) A comparison of one-shot and recovery methods in T1 imaging. Magn Reson Med 7:23-34
23. Gowland P, Mansfield P (1993) Accurate measurement of T1 in vivo in less than 3 seconds using echo-planar imaging. Magn Reson Med 30:351-354
24. Ordidge RJ, Gibbs P, Chapman B et al (1990) High-speed multislice T1 mapping using inversion-recovery echo-planar imaging. Magn Reson Med 16:238-245
25. Clare S, Jezzard P (2001) Rapid T(1) mapping using multislice echo planar imaging. Magn Reson Med 45:630-634
26. Gowland PA, Leach MO (1991) A simple method for the restoration of signal polarity in multi-image inversion recovery sequences for measuring T1. Magn Reson Med 18:224-231
27. Parry A, Clare S, Jenkinson M et al (2002) White matter and lesion T1 relaxation times increase in parallel and correlate with disability in multiple sclerosis. J Neurol 249:1279-1286
28. Griffin CM, Chard DT, Parker GJ et al (2002) The relationship between lesion and normal appearing brain tissue abnormalities in early relapsing remitting multiple sclerosis. J Neurol 249:193-199
29. Vaithianathar L, Tench CR,Morgan PS, Constantinescu CS (2003) Magnetic resonance imaging of the cervical spinal cord in multiple sclerosis – a quantitative T1 relaxation time mapping approach. J Neurol 250:307-315
30. Vaithianathar L, Tench CR, Morgan PS (2002) T1 relaxation time mapping of white matter tracts in multiple sclerosis defined by diffusion tensor imaging. J Neurol 249:1272-1278
31. Nusbaum AO, Tang CY, Wei T (2000) Whole-brain diffusion MR histograms differ between MS subtypes. Neurology 54:1421-1427
32. Fu L, Matthews PM, De Stefano N et al (1998) Imaging axonal damage of normal-appearing white matter in multiple sclerosis. Brain 121:103-113

33. Sarchielli P, Presciutti O, Pelliccioli GP et al (1999) Absolute quantification of brain metabolites by proton magnetic resonance spectroscopy in normal-appearing white matter of multiple sclerosis patients. Brain 122:513-521
34. Feinstein A, Kartsounis LD, Miller DH et al (1992) Clinically isolated lesions of the type seen in multiple sclerosis: a cognitive, psychiatric and MRI follow up study. J Neurol Neurosurg Psyhciatry 55:869-876
35. Miller DH, Grossman RI, Reingold SC, McFarland HF (1998) The role of magnetic resonance techniques in understanding and managing multiple sclerosis. Brain 121:3-24
36. Trapp BD, Peterson J, Ransohoff RM et al (1998) Axonal transection in the lesions of multiple sclerosis. N Engl J Med 338:278-285
37. Ferguson B, Matyszak MK, Esiri MM, Perry VH (1997) Axonal damage in acute multiple sclerosis lesions. Brain 120:393-399
38. Losseff NA, Miller DH (1998) Measures of brain and spinal cord atrophy in multiple sclerosis. J Neurol Neurosurg Psychiatry 64 (Suppl 1):S102-S105
39. Matthews PM (1999) Axonal loss and demyelation in multiple sclerosis. J Neurol Neurosurg Psychiatry 67:708-709
40. Foong J, Rozewicz L, Chong WK (2000) A comparison of neuropsychological deficits in primary and secondary progressive multiple sclerosis. J Neurol 247:97-101
41. Leary SM, Davie CA, Parker GJ et al (1999) 1H magnetic resonance spectroscopy of normal appearing white matter in primary progressive multiple sclerosis. J Neurol 246:1023-1026
42. Evangelou N, Konz D, Esiri MM et al (2000) Regional axonal loss in the corpus callosum correlates with cerebral white matter lesion volume and distribution in multiple sclerosis. Brain 123:1845-1849
43. Nieuwenhuys R, Voogd J, van Huijzen C (1981) The human central nervous system. A synopsis and atlas. Springer, Berlin Heidelberg New York, pp 163-168
44. Parry A, Clare S, Jenkinson M et al (2003) MRI brain T1 relaxation time changes in MS patients increase over time in both the white matter and the cortex. J Neuroimaging 13:234-239
45. Filippi M, Rocca MA, Martino G et al (1998) Magnetization transfer changes in the normal appearing white matter precede the appearance of enhancing lesions in patients with multiple sclerosis. Ann Neurol 43:809-814
46. Goodkin DE, Rooney WD, Sloan R et al (1998) A serial study of new MS lesions and the white matter from which they arise. Neurology 51:1689-1697
47. Werring DJ, Brassat D, Droogan AG et al (2000) The pathogenesis of lesions and normal-appearing white matter changes in multiple sclerosis: a serial diffusion MRI study. Brain 123:1667-1676
48. Lee MA, Smith S, Palace J, Matthews PM (1998) Defining multiple sclerosis disease activity using MRI T2-weighted difference imaging. Brain 121:2095-2102
49. Qian ZM, Shen X (2001) Brain iron transport and neurodegeneration. Trends Mol Med 7:103-108
50. Bakshi R, Dmochowski J, Shaikh ZA, Jacobs L (2001) Grey matter T2 hypointensity is related to plaques and atrophy in the brains of multiple sclerosis patients. J Neurol Sci 185:19-26
51. Drayer B, Burger P, Hurwitz B et al (1987) Reduced signal intensity on MR images of thalamus and putamen in multiple sclerosis: increased iron content? AJR Am J Roentgenol 149:357-363
52. Grimaud J, Millar J, Thorpe JW et al (1995) Signal intensity on MRI of basal ganglia in multiple sclerosis. J Neurol Neurosurg Psychiatry 59:306-308
53. Bakshi R, Shaikh ZA, Janardhan V (2000) MRI T2 shortening ('black T2') in multiple sclerosis: frequency, location, and clinical correlation. Neuroreport 11:15-21

54. Barnes D, McDonald WI, Johnson G et al (1987) Quantitative nuclear magnetic resonance imaging: characterisation of experimental cerebral oedema. J Neurol Neurosurg Psychiatry 50:125-133
55. Barnes D, McDonald WI, Landon DN, Johnson G (1988) The characterization of experimental gliosis by quantitative nuclear magnetic resonance imaging. Brain 111:83-94
56. van Walderveen MA, Lycklama GJ, Ader HJ et al (2001) Hypointense lesions on T1-weighted spin-echo magnetic resonance imaging: relation to clinical characteristics in subgroups of patients with multiple sclerosis. Arch Neurol 58:76-81
57. van Walderveen MA, Truyen L, van Oosten BV et al (1999) Development of hypointense lesions on T1-weighted spin-echo magnetic resonance images in multiple sclerosis: relation to inflammatory activity. Arch Neurol 56:345-351
58. Lucchinetti C, Brück W, Parisi J et al (2000) Heterogeneity of multiple sclerosis lesions: implications for the pathogenesis of demyelination. Ann Neurol 47:707-717

Chapter 7

Diffusion-Weighted Imaging of the Normal-Appearing White Matter in Multiple Sclerosis

M. Rovaris, M. Filippi

Introduction

Conventional magnetic resonance (MR) imaging (MRI) is widely used for the diagnosis of multiple sclerosis (MS), because of its ability to demonstrate the presence of central nervous system (CNS) lesions with dissemination in space and time [1]. In addition, when monitoring the evolution of MS, serial brain MRI scans may disclose the occurrence of disease activity and the accumulation of disease burden with a greater sensitivity than the clinical assessment of relapses and neurological disability. Nevertheless, since a clear discrepancy between clinical and conventional MRI findings in patients with established MS has emerged from most of the available studies [2], there is an urgent need for more accurate neuroimaging techniques to monitor MS evolution.

Diffusion-weighted imaging (DWI) is a quantitative, MR-based technique potentially useful for the study of MS, thanks to its increased pathological specificity over conventional MRI and its ability to assess in vivo the presence of tissue damage occurring outside T_2-visible lesions, i.e. in the so-called normal-appearing white (NAWM) and grey (NAGM) matter. It is well known from postmortem studies that MS pathology does not spare white matter regions which appear normal on a macroscopic examination [3, 4]. MS-related NAWM abnormalities include various pathological substrates, ranging from inflammatory infiltrates to loss of myelin and axons, seem to occur at least partially independently of the burden of macroscopic, MRI-visible lesions [5], and their extent and severity might account for the development of irreversible disability in patients with progressive MS [6]. This chapter summarizes the contribution of DWI to the quantification and characterization of MS-related NAWM damage, with the ultimate aims of providing new insights into the pathobiology of the disease and reviewing the potential use of DWI as a paraclinical tool to monitor MS evolution.

DWI and NAWM Study: Physical Basis and Methodological Aspects

Diffusion is defined as the microscopic random translational motion of molecules in a fluid system. In the central nervous system (CNS), diffusion is influenced by the microstructural components of tissue, including cell membranes and organelles. The diffusion coefficient of biological tissues (which can be measured in vivo by MRI) is, therefore, lower than the diffusion coefficient in free water and it is named "apparent diffusion coefficient" (ADC) [7]. Pathological processes which modify tissue integrity, thus resulting in a loss or increased permeability of "restricting" barriers, can cause an increase of the ADC values. Since some cellular structures are aligned on the scale of an MR image pixel, the measurement of diffusion is also dependent on the direction in which diffusion is measured. As a consequence, diffusion measurements can give information about the size, shape, integrity, and geometry of tissues [8]. A measure of diffusion which is independent on the orientation of structures is provided by the mean diffusivity $\bar{D}$, the average of the ADCs measured in three orthogonal directions. A full characterization of diffusion can be obtained in terms of a tensor [9], a 3×3 matrix which accounts for the correlation existing between molecular displacement along orthogonal directions. From the tensor, it is possible to derive $\bar{D}$, equal to one-third of its trace, and some other dimensionless indices of anisotropy. One of the most used of these indices is fractional anisotropy (FA) [10, 11], which represents a measure of intravoxel fiber coherence. More recently, an index of intervoxel coherence (C), which represents the degree of similarity of orientation of adjacent voxels, has also been proposed [12]. Clearly, MS-related pathological changes (e.g., demyelination and axonal loss) have the potential to modify the integrity and permeability of biological barriers limiting molecular motion in the living brain, thus leading to DWI-detectable quantitative changes reflecting the extent of tissue damage in MS.

In the vast majority of available MS studies, the analysis of DWI data has been conducted either on a region-of-interest (ROI) or on a histogram-based approach. ROI analysis enables detailed information on the DWI characteristics of clinically eloquent NAWM sites, such as the internal capsule and the corpus callosum, to be obtained. Using histogram analysis, information related to the status of specific brain structures is inevitably lost. However, the amount of operator intervention is reduced, thus limiting both the measurement variability in serial studies and the time needed for the analysis [13]. In addition, the recent development of fully automated techniques to segment the various components of brain parenchyma has enabled us to obtain histograms of diffusivity values from the NAWM in isolation, by preliminarily excluding from the analysis those pixels belonging to T_2-visible lesions or grey matter. The latter approach seems to be accurate and reproducible [14, 15] and is currently being applied to the study of many neurological conditions.

DWI and NAWM Damage: Cross-Sectional Studies

ROI-Based Studies

Numerous DWI studies of MS have consistently shown that ADC or $\bar{D}$ values of NAWM are higher than those of white matter from healthy controls, but lower than those measured in T_2-visible MS lesions [12, 14, 16-31]. Studies with diffusion tensor imaging (DTI) showed that FA values of NAWM are lower than those of corresponding white matter from controls and higher than those of T_2-visible lesions [14, 20, 21, 25, 28, 29]. The values of C were also found to be significantly reduced in ROI from the parietal pericallosal areas of MS patients compared to those of healthy controls [12]. Only one study by Griffin et al. [32], which was conducted in a group of 28 patients with early relapsing-remitting (RR) MS (recruited within 3 years from the clinical onset of the disease) did not find any significant differences in diffusivity and anisotropy values of NAWM regions between patients and controls. A preliminary study of patients at presentation with clinically isolated syndrome (CIS) suggestive of MS [33] also failed to detect significant differences between NAWM ADC values from patients and those from healthy controls.

DWI studies assessing changes in different brain regions showed that NAWM abnormalities in MS are widespread, but tend to be more severe in sites where MRI-visible MS lesions are usually located [12, 14, 21, 25, 28] and in periplaque regions [34, 35]. In the study by Filippi et al. [28], NAWM diffusivity and anisotropy values differed between MS patients and controls only for periventricular and frontal lobe white matter regions. Intriguingly, however, when data from the subgroup of patients with primary progressive (PP) MS were considered in isolation, significant DWI changes were also found in the internal capsule and corpus callosum [28], which might contribute to explaining, at least partially, the locomotor and cognitive impairment seen in these patients [35].

Histogram-Based Studies

The average $\bar{D}$ measured in a large portion of brain NAWM was found to be significantly higher than that of healthy controls [14]. In a recent, large-scale study [37], NAWM $\bar{D}$ and FA histogram-derived metrics were found to be significantly different between PPMS patients and healthy subjects. Interestingly, whereas average $\bar{D}$ values were significantly higher in secondary progressive (SP) than in PP MS patients, NAWM FA histogram-derived quantities did not significantly differ between the two patients' groups. These findings confirm that, in PPMS patients, NAWM is not spared by the MS pathological processes, even though it is involved to a lesser degree than in the SP form of the disease, and that these MRI-indetectable changes might contribute to the accumulation of irreversible neurological deficits. Less pronounced but significant changes of NAWM diffusivity have also been described in another histogram-based study of patients with early-onset MS [38], which is traditionally considered a less severe form of the disease. On the other hand, NAWM $\bar{D}$ and FA histogram-derived quantities did not differ between healthy subjects and patients with established MS and non-specific findings on conventional MRI scans of the brain [39]. Inglese et al. [40] found no significant abnormalities of water diffusion in the normal-appearing brain tissue of patients with acute disseminated encephalomyelitis (ADEM), who were scanned after an average of 2 years from the clinical onset of the disease. The latter data can not rule out that reversible changes may occur in the NAWM during the acute phase of ADEM, but they show that, unlike what happens in MS, brain tissue outside residual MRI-visible lesions seems to be spared by ADEM.

Correlations Between DWI and Other MRI-Derived Quantities

DWI changes in the NAWM have been reported to correlate with the burden of MRI-visible lesions [14, 21, 22, 28, 31, 33, 41, 42], but the average magnitude of the observed correlations was only moderate. These correlations were found to be stronger for patients with CIS [33] and when the lesion load of individual cerebral lobes was correlated with diffusivity and anisotropy values in the corresponding callosal regions [31]. The magnitude of the correlation between DTI-derived metrics reflecting water diffusivity and those reflecting tissue anisotropy in the NAWM is also highly variable from one study to another [12, 28, 29], being always moderate at best. This suggests that the study of water diffusivity and anisotropy can provide complementary information, but also that MS tissue damage may affect DTI-derived indices differently in accordance with the heterogeneous aspects of NAWM pathology.

DWI and NAWM Damage: Longitudinal Studies

Two different ROI-based DWI studies consistently detected increased $\bar{D}$ values in NAWM areas subsequently involved by new, T_2-visible MS lesions [23, 24], suggesting that focal vasogenic edema and demyelination beyond the resolution of conventional MRI can play a part in the NAWM changes preceding new lesion formation in MS. A 1-year longitudinal study of DWI changes in the NAWM of CIS patients [33] found that ADC values become significantly higher than those of healthy controls only on follow-up scans, and that they are significantly correlated with T_2-hyperintense lesion load at the same timepoint. Considering that the vast majority (84%) of these patients also had MRI evidence of spatial and temporal disease dissemination, thus fulfilling the criteria for MS diagnosis [1], these findings indicate that DWI is sensitive to the appearance of NAWM changes from the earliest phase of the disease.

In a preliminary study [43] of 26 untreated patients with RRMS who underwent conventional MRI and DTI scans every 3 months for 18 months, NAWM and NAGM diffusivity and anisotropy histograms were produced for a large portion of the brain. A significant decrease of average NAGM FA and a significant increase of average NAGM $\bar{D}$ and brain T_2-hyperintense lesion load were observed over the study period, whereas no significant changes were found for NAWM $\bar{D}$ and FA histogram-derived quantities. In another longitudinal study [44], 54 PPMS and 22 SPMS patients underwent conventional MRI and DTI at baseline and after 1 year. None of these patients' groups showed significant changes of

NAWM histogram-derived quantities over the follow-up period, whereas a significant increase of lesion diffusivity and decrease of NAGM FA were seen.

Findings from histogram-based longitudinal DWI studies are, therefore, in apparent contrast to those of other ROI-based studies of small groups of RRMS patients. For instance, Werring et al. [24] found an estimated rate of 1.4% increase per month for diffusivity values in 19 NAWM regions which remained unaffected by T_2-visible lesions over a period of 1 year. One possible explanation for the negative results of histogram-based DWI studies is that, by computing an average of the diffusivity values from the whole of the NAWM, sensitivity to longitudinal changes occurring in some regions may have been lost. This may happen because the pathological substrates underlying the accumulation of MS brain damage may lead to opposite changes of diffusivity values. Demyelination and axonal loss are expected to provoke a loss of restricting barriers to water molecular motion, i.e., an increase of $\bar{D}$ values. On the other hand, gliosis and cytotoxic edema may decrease the diffusivity of free water and, therefore, reduce the corresponding $\bar{D}$ values from diseased brain tissues.

DWI and the Pathobiology of NAWM Damage in MS

DWI results just indicate a disorganization of structural barriers to water molecular motion in the NAWM, but the possible pathological substrates of these findings have not yet been fully defined. Diffuse astrocytic hyperplasia, patchy edema, perivascular infiltration, gliosis, abnormally thin myelin, and axonal loss are all known to occur in the NAWM of patients with MS [3]. While all these processes might reduce FA, myelin and axonal loss should lead to increased water diffusivity. As a consequence, these latter pathological changes are the most likely contributors to the increased water diffusivity and decreased FA observed in the NAWM. However, it is worth remembering that diffusivity and anisotropy can be differently affected by other substrates of MS pathology, such as reactive gliosis, that may on the one hand cause a partial restriction of molecular diffusivity while on the other provoking a concomitant decrease of tissue anisotropy due to the loss of fiber organization. The average, modest magnitude of the observed correlations between the severity of diffusivity changes of the NAWM and that of MRI-visible MS lesions, as well as their relatively weak relationship with conventional MRI-detectable lesion burden, indicate that NAWM changes are not merely the result of Wallerian degeneration of axons traversing larger lesions, but they may also reflect small focal abnormalities beyond the resolution of conventional scanning.

DWI Studies of NAWM Damage: Clinical Correlations

Several cross-sectional studies [12, 21, 22, 28, 37] did not find significant correlations between the average NAWM diffusivity or anisotropy values and the severity of MS neurological disability, as assessed by the Expanded Disability Status Scale (EDSS) [45] score, nor significant differences between MS clinical phenotypes as regards the severity of overall DWI changes in the NAWM [19, 29]. Reasons for these negative findings may include the limited brain coverage of DWI scans [19] and the narrow range of disabilities that was considered by some studies [21, 22], but also the limitations of the EDSS, which is heavily weighted towards locomotor disability and less sensitive to the clinical manifestations of cerebral dysfunction. When the DWI characteristics of clinically eloquent NAWM regions were studied, a significant relationship with patients' EDSS scores was found for corpus callosum and internal capsule FA [12] and for cerebral peduncle $\bar{D}$ and FA [29]. In addition, in a preliminary DWI study of cognitive impairment in patients with RRMS [46], moderate correlations were found between several NAWM histogram-derived DWI quantities and neuropsychological test scores.

Available data from longitudinal DWI studies [33, 43, 44] did not show any predictive value of NAWM DWI characteristics at baseline for the clinical evolution of the disease during the corresponding follow-up periods, nor did they show a significant relationship between the observed changes of DWI and those of clinical findings. Only the study by Caramia et al. [33] reported a significantly higher EDSS score after 1 year of observation for CIS patients with abnormal NAWM diffusivity values on the corresponding DWI studies than for those without such changes. However, this might be due to the relatively short duration of all these studies (ranging between 12 and 18 months), to the limited size of the patient samples and, as already discussed, to the inability of the EDSS to reflect a significant deterioration of cerebral functions.

DWI Studies of NAWM Damage: Future Perspectives

Due to the different tissue anisotropies, DTI is able not only to distinguish white from grey matter [14], but also to elucidate the macroscopic volume-averaged orientation of the microstructure therein. The anisotropy provides the basis of diffusion tensor (DT) tractography methods, developed to determine the pathways of anatomical CNS connections through the white matter in vivo. There are several methodological limitations to DTI that degrade the information about the spatial orientation of fiber tracts which is contained within the DT. These include the poor resolution of DWI data in comparison with the size of fiber tracts, and the low signal-to-noise ratio of the DWI data from which the DT is estimated, which introduces errors in the directional information derived from it. Recently, several authors have developed different tractography techniques that utilize the directional and anisotropy information contained in a given voxel to connect neighboring voxels and to visualize white matter tracts in vivo [47-49]. The development of these methods to identify and segment a single brain tract is important because this would allow a detailed assessment of damage within it, and a subsequent comparison with relevant clinical data. Tench and coworkers [50] used this technique to map the corpus callosum and the pyramidal tracts from 14 MS patients and 10 controls and to measure the corresponding ADC values within these tracts. The ADC was significantly higher in patients than in controls, and it was higher in the corpus callosum than in the pyramidal tracts for both groups.

The application of tractography methods to segment the different functional white matter structures in MS patients might allow the strength of the correlations between clinical and MRI findings to be improved. Wilson et al. [51] produced maps of pyramidal tracts from DTI scans of 25 patients with RRMS and measured the relative anisotropy along these pathways. Significant correlations were found between the latter parameter and patients' EDSS and pyramidal functional system scores, whereas T_2 lesion burden and diffusion histogram parameters did not correlate with clinical findings. Vaithianathar et al. [52] used DTI-based tractography to map the pyramidal tracts in 25 patients with RRMS. Then, they sampled T_1 relaxation time values along the corresponding trajectories on coregistered whole-brain T_1 maps. Pyramidal tract T_1, but not total white matter T_1 values, correlated significantly with the severity of patients' neurological disability. The results of these preliminary studies confirm that white matter tract mapping using DTI is feasible and may increase the sensitivity and specificity of MR-based techniques in the assessment of clinically relevant structural MS pathology.

Newer acquisition schemes for DWI, such as high *b*-value images [53, 54], may further increase the sensitivity of "conventional", low *b*-value DWI in the detection of NAWM abnormalities and therefore provide a more accurate picture of the severity of MS.

Although DWI of the optic nerve and the spinal cord would be desirable to achieve a more complete picture of how MS can affect clinically eloquent white matter pathways in the CNS, DWI in these regions presents a considerable technical challenge [55]. Nevertheless, successful DWI of the optic nerve [56, 57] and spinal cord [58-64] has been recently obtained. One published study assessed water diffusion in the optic nerve of patients with demyelinating optic neuritis [56] and demonstrated significant different optic nerve ADC values between controls and patients. This study also showed that ADC differs between acute and chronic optic neuritis cases: ADC was found to be decreased in the acute (inflammatory) stage of optic neuritis, and increased in the chronic phase. Another study assessed water diffusion in seven cord lesions of three MS patients with locomotor disability [58], reporting that these lesions had higher $\bar{D}$ values than the cord tissue from healthy volunteers.

Conclusions

DWI allows detection and quantification of subtle changes occurring in the NAWM of MS patients, where measures of tissue anisotropy seem to be more sensitive than those of water diffusivity to disease-related tissue damage. Although DWI changes reflect a net loss of structural organization, at present we can only speculate on their possible pathological substrates in the NAWM. Postmortem studies correlating DWI findings with histopathology of MS patients are therefore warranted.

Despite the aforementioned limitations, DWI promises to increase our understanding of the pathobiology of MS-related NAWM damage, including through the investigation of the relationship between DWI metrics and other MR quantities derived from magnetization transfer MRI, MR spectroscopy, and functional MRI. Available data seem to suggest that ROI-based DWI studies of specific areas, rather than histogram-based studies of large portions of the brain, might be helpful to address this issue, with the potential to obtain further insights from the application of tractography techniques.

To investigate the clinical correlates and the prognostic value of DWI-detectable NAWM damage in MS, further studies are needed with large cohorts of patients, long follow-up periods, and reliable and comprehensive clinical measures of disease evolution. Both DT tractography and DWI of the spinal cord have a great potential to increase the utility of diffusion-based MR techniques in the assessment of clinically relevant structural MS pathology.

References

1. McDonald WI, Compston A, Edan G et al (2001) Recommended diagnostic criteria for multiple sclerosis: guidelines from the international panel on the diagnosis of multiple sclerosis. Ann Neurol 50:121-127
2. Filippi M, Grossman RI (2002) MRI techniques to monitor MS evolution: the present and the future. Neurology 58:1147-1153
3. Allen IV, McKeown SR (1979) A histological, histochemical and biochemical study of the macroscopically normal white matter in multiple sclerosis. J Neurol Sci 41:81-91
4. Evangelou N, Esiri MM, Smith S et al (2000) Quantitative pathological evidence for axonal loss in normal appearing white matter in multiple sclerosis. Ann Neurol 47:391-395
5. Evangelou N, Konz D, Esiri MM et al (2000) Regional axonal loss in the corpus callosum correlates with cerebral white matter lesion volume and distribution in multiple sclerosis. Brain 123:1845-1849
6. Filippi M, Tortorella C, Bozzali M (1999) Normal-appearing-white-matter changes in multiple sclerosis: the contribution of magnetic resonance techniques. Mult Scler 5:273-282
7. Le Bihan D, Breton E, Lallemand D et al (1986) MR imaging of intravoxel incoherent motions: application to diffusion and perfusion in neurologic disorders. Radiology 161:401-407
8. Le Bihan D, Turner R, Pekar J, Moonen CTW (1991) Diffusion and perfusion imaging by gradient sensitization: design, strategy and significance. J Magn Reson Imaging 1:7-8
9. Basser PJ, Mattiello J, Le Bihan D (1994) Estimation of the effective self-diffusion tensor from the NMR spin-echo. J Magn Reson B 103:247-254
10. Pierpaoli C, Jezzard P, Basser PJ et al (1996) Diffusion tensor MR imaging of the human brain. Radiology 201:637-648

11. Basser PJ, Pierpaoli C (1996) Microstructural features measured using diffusion tensor imaging. J Magn Reson B 111:209-219
12. Cercignani M, Bozzali M, Iannucci G et al (2002) Intra-voxel and inter-voxel coherence in patients with multiple sclerosis assessed using diffusion tensor MRI. J Neurol 249:875-883
13. Cercignani M, Bammer R, Sormani MP et al (2003) Inter-sequence and inter-imaging unit variability of diffusion tensor MR imaging histogram-derived metrics of the brain in healthy volunteers. AJNR Am J Neuroradiol 24:638-643
14. Cercignani M, Bozzali M, Iannucci G et al (2001) Magnetisation transfer ratio and mean diffusivity of normal appearing white and grey matter from patients with multiple sclerosis. J Neurol Neurosurg Psychiatry 70:311-317
15. Cercignani M, Inglese M, Siger-Zajdel M, Filippi M (2001) Segmenting white matter, grey matter and cerebro-spinal fluid using diffusion tensor MRI-derived indices. Magn Reson Imaging 19:1167-1172
16. Larsson HBW, Thomsen C, Frederiksen J et al (1992) In vivo magnetic resonance diffusion measurement in the brain of patients with multiple sclerosis. Magn Reson Imaging 10:7-12
17. Christiansen P, Gideon P, Thomsen C et al (1993) Increased water self-diffusion in chronic plaques and in apparently normal white matter in patients with multiple sclerosis. Acta Neurol Scand 87:195-199
18. Horsfield MA, Lai M, Webb SL et al (1996) Apparent diffusion coefficients in benign and secondary progressive multiple sclerosis by nuclear magnetic resonance. Magn Reson Med 36:393-400
19. Droogan AG, Clark CA, Werring DJ et al (1999) Comparison of multiple sclerosis clinical subgroups using navigated spin echo diffusion-weighted imaging. Magn Reson Imaging 17:653-661
20. Werring DJ, Clark CA, Barker GJ et al (1999) Diffusion tensor imaging of lesions and normal-appearing white matter in multiple sclerosis. Neurology 52:1626-1632
21. Filippi M, Iannucci G, Cercignani M et al (2000) A quantitative study of water diffusion in multiple sclerosis lesions and normal-appearing white matter using echo-planar imaging. Arch Neurol 57:1017-1021
22. Cercignani M, Iannucci G, Rocca MA et al (2000) Pathologic damage in MS assessed by diffusion-weighted and magnetization transfer MRI. Neurology 54:1139-1144
23. Rocca MA, Cercignani M, Iannucci G et al (2000) Weekly diffusion-weighted imaging of normal-appearing white matter in MS. Neurology 55:882-884
24. Werring DJ, Brassat D, Droogan AG et al (2000) The pathogenesis of lesions and normal-appearing white matter changes in multiple sclerosis. A serial diffusion MRI study. Brain 123:1667-1676
25. Bammer R, Augustin M, Strasser-Fuchs S et al (2000) Magnetic resonance diffusion tensor imaging for characterizing diffuse and focal white matter abnormalities in multiple sclerosis. Magn Reson Med 44:583-59
26. Nusbaum AO, Lu D, Tang CY, Atlas SW (2000) Quantitative diffusion measurements in focal multiple sclerosis lesions: correlations with appearance on T1-weighted MR images. AJR Am J Roentgenol 175:821-825
27. Roychowdhury S, Maldijan JA, Grossman RI (2000) Multiple sclerosis: comparison of trace apparent diffusion coefficients with MR enhancement pattern of lesions. AJNR Am J Neuroradiol 21:869-874
28. Filippi M, Cercignani M, Inglese M et al (2001) Diffusion tensor magnetic resonance imaging in multiple sclerosis. Neurology 56:304-311
29. Ciccarelli O, Werring DJ, Wheeler-Kingshott CA et al (2001) Investigation of MS normal-appearing brain using diffusion tensor MRI with clinical correlations. Neurology 56:926-933
30. Werring DJ, Clark CA, Droogan AG et al (2001) Water diffusion is elevated in wide-

spread regions of normal-appearing white matter in multiple sclerosis and correlates with diffusion in focal lesions. Mult Scler 7:83-89
31. Ciccarelli O, Werring DJ, Barker GJ et al (2003) A study of the mechanisms of normal-appearing white matter damage in multiple sclerosis using diffusion tensor imaging. Evidence of Wallerian degeneration. J Neurol 250:287-292
32. Griffin CM, Chard DT, Ciccarelli O et al (2001) Diffusion tensor imaging in early relapsing-remitting multiple sclerosis. Mult Scler 7:290-297
33. Caramia F, Pantano P, Di Legge S et al (2002) A longitudinal study of MR diffusion changes in normal appearing white matter of patients with early multiple sclerosis. Magn Reson Imaging 20:383-388
34. Guo AC, Jewells VL, Provenzale JM (2001) Analysis of normal-appearing white matter in multiple sclerosis: comparison of diffusion tensor MR imaging and magnetization transfer imaging. AJNR Am J Neuroradiol 22:1893-1900
35. Guo AC, MacFall JR, Provenzale JM (2002) Multiple sclerosis: diffusion tensor MR imaging for evaluation of normal-appearing white matter. Radiology 222:729-736
36. Thompson AJ, Polman CH, Miller DH et al (1997) Primary progressive multiple sclerosis. Brain 120:1085-1096
37. Rovaris M, Bozzali M, Iannucci G et al (2002) Assessment of normal-appearing white and grey matter in patients with primary progressive multiple sclerosis. Arch Neurol 59:1406-1412
38. Mezzapesa DM, Rocca MA, Falini A et al (2004) A preliminary diffusion tensor and magnetization transfer MRI study of early-onset MS. Arch Neurol 61:366-368
39. Rocca MA, Pagani E, Ghezzi A et al (2003) Functional cortical changes in patients with multiple sclerosis and nonspecific findings on conventional magnetic resonance imaging scans of the brain. Neuroimage 19:826-836
40. Inglese M, Salvi F, Iannucci G et al (2002) Magnetization transfer and diffusion tensor MR imaging of acute disseminated encephalomyelitis. AJNR Am J Neuroradiol 23:267-272
41. Cercignani M, Inglese M, Pagani E et al (2001) Mean diffusivity and fractional anisotropy histograms in patients with multiple sclerosis. AJNR Am J Neuroradiol 22:952-958
42. Iannucci G, Rovaris M, Giacomotti L et al (2001) Correlations between measures of multiple sclerosis pathology derived from T2, T1, magnetization transfer and diffusion tensor MR imaging. AJNR Am J Neuroradiol 22:1462-1467
43. Oreja-Guevara C, Rovaris M, Caputo D et al (2003) Short-term evolution of brain tissue damage in untreated relapsing-remitting multiple sclerosis patients: an in vivo study using diffusion tensor MRI [abstract]. Mult Scler 9(Suppl 1):S59
44. Rovaris M, Gallo A, Caputo D et al (2003) Short-term evolution of brain tissue damage in patients with primary progressive multiple sclerosis:an in vivo study using diffusion tensor MRI [abstract]. Mult Scler 9(Suppl 1):S60
45. Kurtzke JF (1983) Rating neurological impairment in multiple sclerosis: an expanded disability status scale (EDSS). Neurology 33:1444-1452
46. Rovaris M, Iannucci G, Falautano M et al (2002) Cognitive dysfunction in patients with mildly disabling relapsing-remitting multiple sclerosis: an exploratory study with diffusion tensor MR imaging. J Neurol Sci 195:103-109
47. Conturo TE, Lori NF, Cull TS et al (1999) Tracking neuronal fiber pathways in the living human brain. Proc Natl Acad Sci U S A 96:10422-10427
48. Mori S, Crain BJ, Chacko VP, van Zijl PC (1999) Three-dimensional tracking of axonal projections in the brain by magnetic resonance imaging. Ann Neurol 45:265-269
49. Mori S, Kaufmann WE, Davatzikos C et al (2002) Imaging cortical association tracts in the human brain using diffusion-tensor-based axonal tracking. Magn Reson Med 47:215-223

50. Tench CR, Morgan PS, Wilson M, Blumhardt LD (2002) White matter mapping using diffusion tensor MRI. Magn Reson Med 47:967-972
51. Wilson M, Tench CR, Morgan PS, Blumhardt LD (2003) Pyramidal tract mapping by diffusion tensor magnetic resonance imaging in multiple sclerosis: improving correlations with disability. J Neurol Neurosurg Psychiatry 74:203-207
52. Vaithianathar L, Tench CR, Morgan PS et al (2002) T1 relaxation time mapping of white matter tracts in multiple sclerosis defined by diffusion tensor imaging. J Neurol 249:1272-1278
53. Assaf Y, Ben-Bashat D, Chapman J et al (2002) High b-value q-space analyzed diffusion-weighted MRI: application to multiple sclerosis. Magn Reson Med 47:115-126
54. Assaf Y, Cohen Y (2000) Assignment of the water slow-diffusing component in the central nervous system using q-space diffusion MRS: implications for fiber tract imaging. Magn Reson Med 43:191-199
55. Clark CA, Werring DJ (2002) Diffusion tensor imaging in spinal cord: methods and applications – a review. NMR Biomed 15:578-586
56. Iwasawa T, Matoba H, Ogi A et al (1997) Diffusion-weighted imaging of the human optic nerve: a new approach to evaluate optic neuritis in multiple sclerosis. Magn Reson Med 38:484-491
57. Wheeler-Kingshott CA, Parker GJM, Symms MR et al (2002) ADC mapping of the human optic nerve: increased resolution, coverage, and reliability with CSF-suppressed ZOOM-EPI. Magn Reson Med 47:24-31
58. Clark CA, Werring DJ, Miller DH (2000) Diffusion imaging of the spinal cord in vivo: estimation of the principal diffusivities and application to multiple sclerosis. Magn Reson Med 43:133-138
59. Ries M, Jones RA, Dousset V, Moonen CTW (2000) Diffusion tensor MRI of the spinal cord. Magn Reson Med 44:884-892
60. Bammer R, Fazekas F, Augustin M et al (2000) Diffusion-weighted MR imaging of the spinal cord. AJNR Am J Neuroradiol 21:587-591
61. Robertson RL, Maier SE, Mulkern RV et al (2000) MR line-scan diffusion imaging of the spinal cord in children. AJNR Am J Neuroradiol 21:1344-1348
62. Wheeler-Kingshott CA, Hickman SJ, Parker GJ et al (2002) Investigating cervical spinal cord structure using axial diffusion tensor imaging. Neuroimage 16:93-102
63. Bammer R, Augustin M, Prokesch RW et al (2002) Diffusion-weighted imaging of the spinal cord: interleaved echo-planar imaging is superior to fast spin-echo. J Magn Reson Imaging 15:364-373
64. Cercignani M, Horsfield MA, Agosta F, Filippi M (2003) Sensitivity-encoded diffusion tensor MR imaging of the cervical cord. AJNR Am J Neuroradiol 24:1254-1256

Chapter 8

The Relevance of Normal-Appearing White Matter Pathology in Multiple Sclerosis

M. MacInnes, D.L. Arnold

Introduction

Although the current dogma is that multiple sclerosis (MS) is a T-cell-mediated inflammatory demyelinating disease, a number of studies have provided evidence to challenge this concept. Data obtained through the use of MR techniques such as magnetic resonance spectroscopy (MRS) and magnetization transfer imaging support the argument that MS could be primarily a degenerative disease in which focal inflammatory lesions occur secondarily. This chapter will focus on some of the evidence that supports this concept.

MRS and *N*-Acetylaspartate

A noninvasive means to assess the brain's chemical pathology, MRS provides a way to investigate neuronal (including axonal and dendritic) pathology that is not observable using conventional MR imaging (MRI). *N*-Acetyl compounds [largely *N*-acetylaspartate (NAA)] produce the most prominent peak. Located exclusively in the neurons and neuronal processes of adult brains [1], NAA density can serve as a marker of neuronal integrity. Therefore, it is a key metabolite for studying pathology associated with MS. NAA is commonly quantified by expressing its concentration relative to creatine (NAA/Cr), and this has been found to be practical in the context of this disease.

Since the relative creatine concentration remains fairly constant, declines in the NAA/Cr ratio are attributed to declines in NAA. Lower relative concentrations of NAA may reflect neuronal dysfunction, loss, and/or dilution resulting from edema. Research has shown that early decreases in NAA may be largely associated with reversible neuronal dysfunction that occurs in the absence of ongoing cell death, while chronic decreases in NAA are more serious as they are accompanied by cellular loss [2].

Relevance of NAWM Pathology in MS

Consistent with other lines of evidence, MRS studies of NAA in vivo have shown that the so-called "normal-appearing white matter" (NAWM) of MS patients is not normal. NAA is decreased not only in lesions, but also in the NAWM [3]. More recently, studies have shown that NAA is also decreased in the cortical grey matter of MS patients [4], and that the abnormality in NAA in NAWM occurs early in the course of the disease and in patients with relatively low T_2-weighted lesion volumes [5]. A recent study of whole brain NAA (WBNAA) concentrations revealed that patients with clinically isolated syndromes suggestive of MS (CIS) had significantly lower relative concentrations of WBNAA than healthy controls [6]. On average, WBNAA concentrations were reduced by 23% without any correlation with either T_2-weighted or T1-weighted lesion volumes [6].

MT Imaging

Magnetization transfer (MT) imaging can also be used to obtain in vivo information on brain chemical pathology that is not observed on conventional MRI. MT imaging reports on the interactions between mobile protons in water and nonmobile protons associated with macromolecules and lipids, ultimately providing information about tissue structure. In brain, changes in MT are strongly correlated with changes in myelin content [7], and therefore to pathological changes in myelin and axons. Thus, MT imaging can provide an indirect measure of structural changes particularly relevant to MS pathology.

The MT ratio (MTR) is a convenient means of quantifying MT and is commonly used.

MTR images are parametric images based on the difference between the MRI signal intensity before and after the application of a radiofrequency pulse that saturates the MRI signal from protons bound to macromolecules. Unfortunately, decreases in MTR may also be caused by an increase in the mobile proton pool, which can occur as a result of inflammation and edema. However, the effect of edema is relatively small compared to the changes in MTR associated with demyelination [7]. MTR changes in NAWM behave in a fashion analogous to those described above for NAA, in that they are diffusely abnormal in NAWM [8] and can be detected early in the course of MS in patients with low lesion volumes (Fig. 1) [5, 6].

Focal, Prelesional Pathology in the Brain's Normal-Appearing Tissues

The observation of focal pathology in NAWM before the appearance of new inflammatory lesions on MRI has provided important new insights into the potential significance of abnormalities in the NAWM. It has also served to highlight the fact that pathology is evolving in MS lesions for some time prior to the appearance of gadolinium enhancement on MRI.

Focal pathology has been observed months to years before lesion formation through the use of MTR imaging and MRS imaging. Pike and colleagues showed

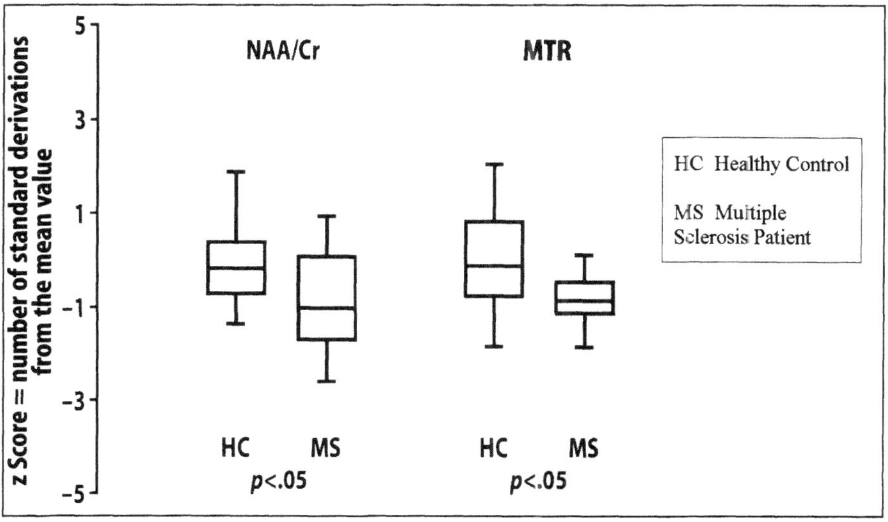

Fig. 1. Box plots showing low NAA/Cr and magnetization transfer ratio (*MTR*) in the brains of MS patients with very low T2-weighted lesion volumes (≤2cc) compared to healthy controls. *NBV*, normalized brain volume; *HC*, healty controls (Adapted from [7])

progressive focal decreases in MTR that antedated lesion formation by years [8]. More recently, Tartaglia and colleagues used ^{1}H-MRS to measure the relative concentration of choline in the NAWM of MS patients [9]. Choline-containing compounds are associated with membrane phospholipids and have been observed at higher levels in association with myelin breakdown such as occurs in acute demyelinating lesions [10]. Serial MRI and MRS revealed that choline levels were significantly higher in areas of NAWM that became lesional on subsequent scans than in areas of NAWM that did not develop lesions [9]. Furthermore, significantly higher choline levels were observed in voxels that displayed increased lesion content on subsequent scans than in voxels whose lesion content had not changed. Focal choline abnormalities were observed even 12 months before lesions became visible on conventional MRI [9].

The prelesional pathology that is present years before lesion appearance appears to accelerate in the months prior to blood-brain barrier breakdown and gadolinium enhancement [11]. Accelerated decreases in MTR were observed just before lesion appearance on conventional MRI [11]. Diffusivity [12], blood volume, and perfusion increase about 1 month prior to blood-brain barrier breakdown and appearance of lesions on MRI [13]. MRS occasionally also reveals release of free lipids from myelin [14]. One may speculate that these short-term changes before the appearance of gadolinium enhancement may reflect low-grade inflammation. The basis for longer-term prelesional changes may be more intriguing as it may not be so simply related to the impending focal inflammatory reaction.

Atrophy

Brain atrophy generally reflects tissue damage and loss of axons, although changes in brain volume can also occur secondary to gliosis, inflammation, edema, changes in hydration status, alcohol, starvation, drugs, etc. Focal axonal injury and loss can be associated with atrophy by a number of different mechanisms. Focal atrophy can result from tissue loss associated with focal axonal injury in lesions. More diffuse atrophy can result from the wallerian degeneration that occurs in distal projection pathways of transected axons [15]. More subtle mechanisms that may be temporally delayed with respect to lesion formation would include a reduced survival time for demyelinated axons that have not been transected and the development of transsynaptic degeneration in neuronal systems [16].

De Stefano and colleagues recently reported significant correlations (r=0.67, p<0.001) between normalized brain volume (NBV) and NAA/Cr [17]. No significant correlations were found between NBV and either T_1-weighted lesion volumes (r=0.3, p=0.2) or T_2-weighted lesion volumes (r=0.4, p<0.1) [17]. The fact that NBV values correlated significantly with NAA/Cr levels and not with lesion volumes suggests that axonal loss is an important contributor to atrophy in the brains of MS patients, and that pathology relevant to atrophy occurs in the normal-appearing tissue rather than in the MRI-visible inflammatory lesions.

Atrophy Occurs at the Earliest Stage of MS

In a group of patients with clinically isolated syndromes suggestive of MS, significant ventricular enlargement occurred over the course of one year in patients who developed MS in that time, compared to those who had no further symptoms [18]. Dalton and colleagues investigated atrophy in early MS and additionally considered its relation to MRI lesion load and/or clinical outcome [19]. In agreement with Brex et al. [18], they saw significant ventricular enlargement in the group of CIS patients who eventually developed MS. Dalton and colleagues also observed that lesions and atrophy appear to be present in patients with CIS who go on to develop MS, but that the correlation between lesions and atrophy was only modest. Again, the weak relationship between atrophy and lesion evolution suggests that atrophy evolves by mechanisms at least partly independent of focal inflammatory activity.

Atrophy Progresses Despite Anti-Inflammatory Therapy

Therapeutic trials that have investigated the effect of immunosuppressive, immunomodulatory agents on atrophy in MS have shed important light onto the relation of atrophy to inflammatory lesions.

In patients with progressive MS, focal inflammatory activity was suppressed by 70-80% following treatment with interferon or with cladribine, but atrophy continued at a rate that was not significantly different from the rate in placebo-treated patients [20-21]. The authors speculated that some of the atrophy in the treated patients may have been due to decreased brain water content resulting from the anti-inflammatory nature of the treatment, but still concluded that the pathology underlying atrophy was not significantly affected by treatment with interferon or cladribine.

Clinical Progression in Secondary Progressive MS Appears to Be Independent of Ongoing Focal Inflammatory Activity

Disability in secondary progressive MS also appears to progress independent of focal inflammatory activity. A study of 1844 MS patients investigated the influence of relapses on progressive disability in MS [22]. Using Kaplan-Meier analyses, Confavreux and colleagues observed that once progressive disability began (defined as reaching an Expanded Disability Status Scale score of 4), the rate at which disability progressed was not affected by relapses that occurred either before onset of the progressive phase or during its course.

Furthermore, Goodkin and colleagues investigated two dosing regimens of interferon β-1b in patients with secondary progressive MS in an attempt to investigate their effects on progressive disability [23]. Under both dosing regimens, relapses were reduced in frequency and duration. The number of new gadolinium-enhancing lesions was also reduced, and a lower progression of T_2-weighted lesion volume was observed. Despite these positive effects, however, the rate of progressive disability in the patients failed to decrease [23].

The fact that disability progresses in MS patients irrespective of the presence or absence of focal inflammatory lesions or relapses, and despite treatment with anti-inflammatory drugs, supports the idea that secondary progression in MS is due to neurodegeneration that progresses at least somewhat independently of inflammation.

Conclusion

This chapter has presented selected examples of relevant research pertaining to the pathology underlying the progression of MS. Increased use of MR techniques such as MT imaging and MRS has provided further insight into the relevance of NAWM pathology. Focal pathology precedes lesion formation. Nonfocal pathology exists throughout the brain in normal-appearing grey and white matter. Brain atrophy and clinical disability both progress apparently independent of the focal inflammatory activity associated with gadolinium enhancement and relapses and are resistant to suppression by anti-inflammatory therapies. Taken together, these findings indicate that MS may not be a primarily inflammatory disease. Rather, MS could be a disease of neural degeneration in which inflammation occurs as a secondary event.

References

1. Simmons ML, Frondoza CG, Coyle JT (1991) Immunocytochemical localization of *N*-acetyl-aspartate with monoclonal antibodies. Neuroscience 45:37-45
2. Dautry C, Vaufrey F, Brouillet E et al (2000) Early *N*-acetylaspartate depletion is a marker of neuronal dysfunction in rats and primates chronically treated with the mitochondrial toxin 3-nitropropionic acid. J Cereb Blood Flow Metab 20:789-799
3. Fu L, Matthews PM, De Stefano N et al (1998) Imaging axonal damage of normal-appearing white matter in multiple sclerosis. Brain 121:103-113
4. Kapeller P, McLean MA, Griffin CM et al (2001) Preliminary evidence for neuronal damage in cortical grey matter and normal appearing white matter in short duration relapsing-remitting multiple sclerosis: a quantitative MR spectroscopic imaging study. J Neurol 248:131-138
5. De Stefano N, Narayanan S, Francis S et al (2002) Diffuse axonal and tissue injury in patients with multiple sclerosis with low cerebral lesion load and no disability. Arch Neurol 59:1565-1571
6. Filippi M, Bozzali M, Rovaris M et al (2003) Evidence for widespread axonal damage at the earliest clinical stage of multiple sclerosis. Brain 126:433-437
7. Dousset V, Grossman RI, Ramer KN et al (1992) Experimental allergic encephalomyelitis and multiple sclerosis: lesion characterization with magnetization transfer imaging. Radiology 182:483-491
8. Pike GB, De Stefano N, Narayanan S et al (1999) Combined magnetization transfer and proton spectroscopic imaging in the assessment of pathologic brain lesions in multiple sclerosis. AJNR Am J Neuroradiol 20:829-837
9. Tartaglia MC, Narayanan S, De Stefano N et al (2002) Choline is increased in pre-lesional normal appearing white matter in multiple sclerosis. J Neurol 249:1382-1390
10. Arnold DL, Matthews PM, Francis GS et al (1992) Proton magnetic resonance spectroscopic imaging for metabolic characterization of demyelinating plaques. Ann Neurol 31:235-241
11. Laule C, Vavasour IM, Whittall KP et al (2003) Evolution of focal and diffuse magnetisation transfer abnormalities in multiple sclerosis. J Neurol 250:924-931
12. Rocca MA, Cercignani M, Iannucci G et al (2000) Weekly diffusion-weighted imaging of normal-appearing white matter in MS. Neurology 55:882-884
13. Wuerfel J, Bellmann-Strobl J, Brunecker P et al (2004) Changes in cerebral perfusion precede plaque formation in multiple sclerosis: a longitudinal perfusion MRI study. Brain 127:111-119
14. Wolinsky J, Narayana P, Fenstermacher M (1990) Proton magnetic resonance spectroscopy in multiple sclerosis. Neurology 40:1764-1769
15. Miller DH, Barkhof F, Frank JA et al (2002) Measurement of atrophy in multiple sclerosis: pathological basis, methodological aspects and clinical relevance. Brain 125:1676-1695
16. Trapp BD, Bö L, Mork S, Chang A (1999) Pathogenesis of tissue injury in MS lesions. J Neuroimmunol 98:49-56
17. De Stefano N, Iannucci G, Sormani MP et al (2002) MR correlates of cerebral atrophy in patients with multiple sclerosis. J Neurol 249:1072-1077
18. Brex PA, Jenkins R, Fox NC et al (2000) Detection of ventricular enlargement in patients at the earliest clinical stage of MS. Neurology 54:1689-1691

19. Dalton CM, Brex PA, Jenkins R et al (2002) Progressive ventricular enlargement in patients with clinically isolated syndromes is associated with the early development of multiple sclerosis. J Neurol Neurosurg Psychiatry 73:141-147
20. Molyneux PD, Kappos L, Polman C et al (2000) The effect of interferon beta-1b treatment on MRI measures of cerebral atrophy in secondary progressive multiple sclerosis. European Study Group on Interferon beta-1b in secondary progressive multiple sclerosis. Brain 123:2256-2263
21. Filippi M, Rovaris M, Iannucci G et al (2000) Whole brain volume changes in patients with progressive MS treated with cladribine. Neurology 55:1714-1718
22. Confavreux C, Vukusic S, Moreau T, Adeleine P (2000) Relapses and progression of disability in multiple sclerosis. N Engl J Med 343:1430-1438
23. Goodkin DE (2000) The North American Study Group on Interferon β-1b in Secondary Progressive MS. Interferon β-1b in secondary progressive multiple sclerosis: clinical and MRI results of a 3-year randomized controlled trial. Neurology 54 (suppl):2352 [Abstract]

NORMAL-APPEARING GREY MATTER

Chapter 9

Grey Matter Pathology in Multiple Sclerosis

B.P. Brink, S.J. Mork, P. van der Valk, L. Bo

Introduction

Multiple sclerosis (MS) is a CNS disease histopathologically characterized by discrete areas of myelin, oligodendrocyte, and axonal loss [1]. The etiology of MS is unknown, but environmental factors and multiple separate genetic loci contribute to disease susceptibility. MS lesions may occur in all CNS parenchymal areas; the predilection sites include the optic nerve, brainstem, spinal cord, periventricular white matter, and subcortical areas. Although MS is frequently called a white matter disease, there is also myelin in grey matter, and grey matter demyelination is extensive in chronic MS [2-7]. This was evidenced even in early pathology studies, using histochemical staining methods for myelin detection [8-11]. The extent of cortical demyelination in MS has been studied in vivo using MRI and post mortem using histochemical or immunohistochemical techniques. Conventional MRI techniques may not be sensitive for cortical lesions, however: in a comparison of postmortem MRI and histological examinations, only 2 of 14 histologically detectable cortical lesions were detected by MRI [3]. In another, similar study none of the 39 cortical plaques identified histologically were detected by MRI, while in periventricular areas the maximum possible number of lesions detected by MRI often exceeded the number of histological plaques [12]. A recent study found a low sensitivity of MRI for purely cortical lesions compared with the grey matter part of combined white matter/grey matter lesions [7]. MRI sensitivity for deep grey matter lesions was slightly higher, at 10%-15% [7, 12]. The reasons for the low sensitivity of conventional MRI could be (1) that the relaxation times of grey matter on T_2-weighted images are close to the relaxation times of MS lesions, (2) partial volume effects due to the proximity to the CSF, and (3) less inflammation and edema in the grey matter lesions [3]. "Normal-appearing grey matter" on MRI thus represents what proves histopathologically to be a mixture of grey matter lesions and nonlesional tissue. This makes it difficult to characterize the clinical significance of grey matter lesions by MRI. Nevertheless, the presence and extent of "juxtacortical" MS lesions on MRI have been correlated with cognitive loss, depression, and epilepsy [13-17].

The sensitivity for cortical lesions is low also by standard histochemical staining techniques on autopsy tissue, such as luxol fast blue [5, 18]. The low MRI and histopathology sensitivity is the likely reason for the paucity of studies on grey matter pathology in MS. The aim of this review is to give a short summary of what is currently known about the extent, distribution, and histopathology of grey matter changes in MS.

Extent and Distribution of Grey Matter MS Lesions

In several early pathology studies MS cases with very extensive cortical demyelination were described. Sander (1898), Dinkler (1904), Schob (1907), and Dawson (1916) reported MS cases with extensive cortical demyelination; in some the majority of lesions were cortical. Large subpial superficial lesions as well as frequent wedge-shaped, round or oval cortical demyelinated areas are described [8-11].

In 1970, Lumsden described frequent involvement of the cerebral cortex in MS, 93.5% of MS cases had cortical lesions at autopsy. In ten "early and severe" MS cases, 280 lesions, constituting 59% of total brain lesions 1-10 mm in diameter, were found to affect the cerebral cortex [19]. This constituted approximately 0.43 plaques per gram wet weight, as compared to 0.26 plaques per gram wet weight in centrum ovale and corpus callosum (excluding the immediate periventricular zone). There was regional variation, with the highest extent of demyelination in the superior frontal, anterior central, posterior central, and superior temporal gyrus. In a study by Brownell and Hughes [2], 26% of hemisphere lesions were found to affect grey matter, 17% were at the border between white matter and the cortex, 5% were intracortical, and 4% were in central grey matter.

In a 1999 study of coronal tissue sections from 12 MS brains, Kidd et al. found 478 cortical lesions, 24% of which were intracortical [3]. By histological examination of one case also examined by MRI, it was found that 14 lesions were cortical and 108 lesions juxtacortical; these figures represented 4.3% and 32.9% of the total number of lesions, respectively. Cortical lesions were found to correspond to cortical venular territories, with the possible exception of the largest cortical lesions, which were thought to arise from a series of principal veins, most likely representing the larger collecting central vein of the gyrus.

We studied the extent and distribution of grey matter demyelination in MS by myelin basic protein (MBP) immunohistochemistry, in brain material from 20 chronic MS patients, obtained at autopsy [5]. Four areas were collected from each brain, irrespective of the presence of any macroscopic signs of pathology. Myelinated fibers were organized in three patterns – radial fibers, oblique fibers, and horizontal fibers – in normally myelinated cortices of both MS and control patients. As described previously, the highest density of myelin staining was found in cortical layers 4-6, intermediate density of myelin staining was present in layer 3, and in layers 1 and 2 the density of staining was low [20]. Cortical lesions were classified according to a descriptive system similar to that employed in previous studies [4, 11]. Four different types of cortical lesion were identified on the basis of lesion distribution within cerebral cortex/subcortical white matter. Lesions that extended across both white matter and grey matter were termed type 1 lesions (Fig. 1A). The center of these lesions would often be in the white matter. Subcortical white matter lesions in general did not respect the cortical/white matter border. Lesions within the cerebral cortex that did not extend to the surface of the brain or to the subpial white matter were classified as type 2; these lesions were frequently small (Fig. 1B). The most common cortical lesion type, affecting the largest cortical area, was subpial (type 3) (Figs. 1C, 2A, C); 60% of the cortical lesions were subpial, accounting for 67% of the total cortical demyelinated area. A common appearance of type 3 lesions was long ribbons of subpial demyelination, often affecting several adjacent gyri (Fig. 2A, C). Another appearance of type 3 lesions would be a wedge-shaped lesion, with the base on the surface of the brain. A combination of these patterns, with wedge-like lesion areas within bands of more superficial subpial demyelination, was often present. Lesions that extended throughout the full width of the cerebral cortex without reaching into the subcortical white matter were classified as type 4 (Figs. 1D, 2B, D, H). Type 4 lesions had a striking selectivity for the cerebral cortex, as the border of the lesions often corresponded for long stretches to the white matter/grey matter border (Figs. 1D, 2D). This may lead to almost total demyelination of some gyri without demyelination of the subpial grey matter (Figs. 1D, 2D).

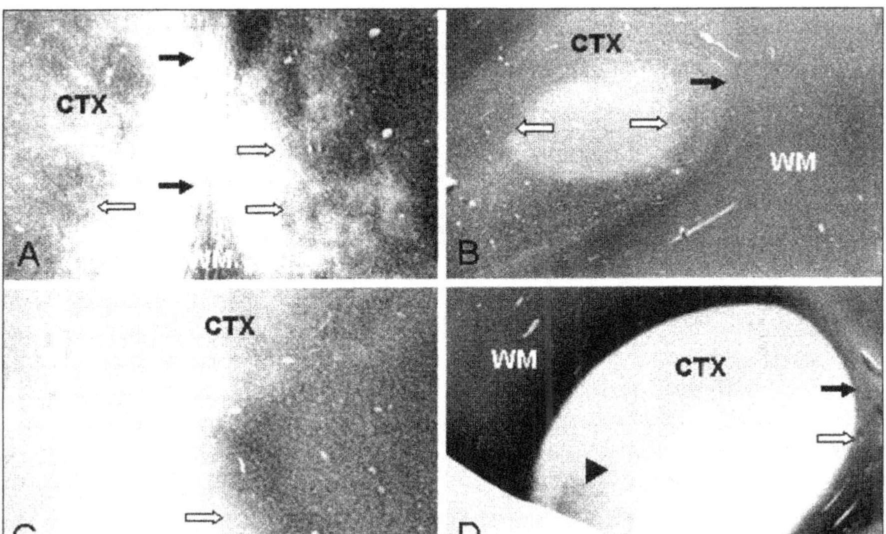

Fig. 1 A-D. Classification of cortical lesions based on lesion location/distribution. Paraffin sections from MS brain stained with anti-MBP (myelin basic protein) antibody. Type 1 lesions (**A**) extend through both white (*WM*) and grey (*CTX*) matter. Type 2 lesions (**B**) are intracortical with no contact with white matter or with the surface of the brain. Type 3 lesions (**C**) extend inward from the surface of the brain, and type 4 lesions (**D**) extend through the whole width of the cortex without reaching into white matter. A small area of probable remyelination is observed (*arrowhead*). *Filled arrows*, border between cerebral cortex and white matter; *open arrows*, border of lesion. Reproduced with permission from the Journal of Neuropathology and Experimental Neurology [5]

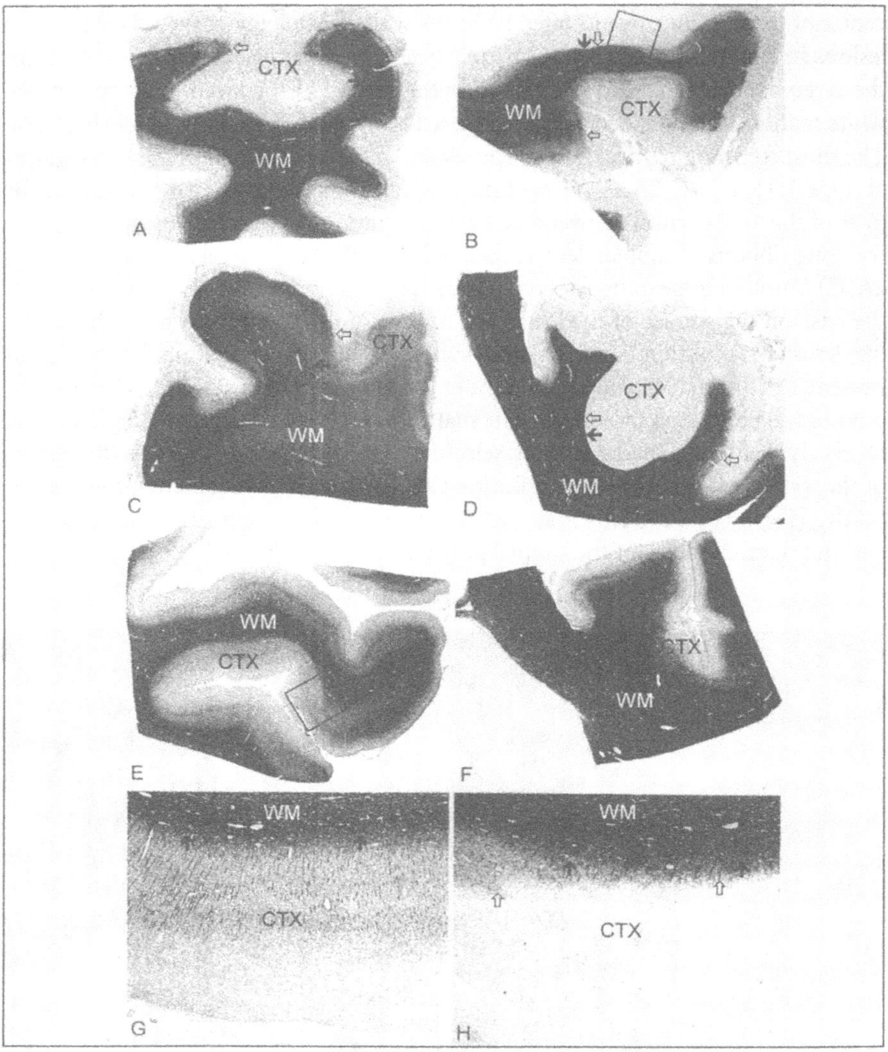

Fig. 2. Paraffin sections immunohistochemically stained with anti-MBP antibody and lightly counterstained with hematoxylin, from a MS patient (**A-D, H**), and a control patient (**E-G**). **A** is from the frontal lobe, **B** and **E** are from the temporal lobe, **C** is from the parietal lobe, and **D** and **F** are from the cingulate gyrus. The MS patient had extensive subpial demyelination in all four tissue specimens (**A-D**), and was thus considered to have general cortical subpial demyelination (GSD). In **A** and **C** the lesion is subpial, but does not span the full width of the cerebral cortex (type 3 lesion). In **B** and **D** the lesion spans the full width of the cortex without reaching into subcortical white matter (type 4 lesion). The cingulate gyrus specimens include periventricular white matter and white matter of the corpus callosum (**D, F**). **G, H** Higher-magnification images from **B** and **E** (*boxes*) shows myelin staining throughout the width of control cerebral cortex (**G**) and subpial demyelination in the MS cortex (**H**). *Open arrows* indicate the lesion border, *filled arrows* delineate the white matter/cerebral cortex border. Reproduced with permission from the Journal of Neuropathology and Experimental Neurology [5]

In 5 of the 20 MS patients studied, subpial demyelination was extensive in all four of the widely spaced tissue blocks selected, indicating a widespread superficial loss of cortical myelin. This was termed *general cortical subpial demyelination* (GSD) (Fig. 2A-D). The cortices of these patients harbored both type 3 and type 4 lesions (Fig. 2A-D). In patients with GSD, cortical lesions affected a mean of 56.6% of the total cortical area examined, as compared to 17.9% in the other MS patients (p<0.001). The mean percentage of demyelinated area in the white matter was 2.2% (median 1.9%) in the GSD patients, which was lower than in the other MS patients (mean 7.9%, median 2.3%), but this difference was not statistically significant (p=0.20).

Histopathology of the Grey Matter in MS

Neuronal Pathology

The histopathology of grey matter MS lesions has been far less extensively studied than white matter lesions, and we are not aware of any studies specifically addressing the pathology of normal-appearing grey matter in MS. In the early twentieth century several investigators presented studies on neuronal pathology in grey matter MS lesions. Dinkler in 1904 described a case of MS where the majority of lesions lay in the cortex of the brain [9]. Demyelination and axonal loss were observed in these lesions. Degenerating neuronal cells surrounded by nests of glial cells were found both in lesions and in nondemyelinated adjoining tissue. A thorough examination of grey matter MS pathology is provided by Dawson, who found that cellular changes were often slight, to such an extent that lesions were not detectable except with a myelin stain [11]. Apart from a complete absence of myelin, frequently no other change was found. Neuronal and axonal changes were often absent, but there were also areas of axonal and neuronal pathology. In such areas neuronal degeneration and atrophy were observed. More cellular changes were found in the deeper layers of the cortex, with fewer changes above layer 4. A glial cell reaction was detected in areas of neuronal degeneration. In lesions confined to the cortex, cellular changes were not nearly so marked. Still, axonal dilatation and neuronal degeneration were also observed in purely cortical areas. Neuronal changes involved chromatolysis, thickened, weakly stained, or absent dendrites, and rounded contour of neurons, not only in the lesion but also in adjoining stretches of cortex.

Peterson et al. studied the presence and extent of neuronal changes in grey matter lesions in material from seven MS patients [4]. In most cortical lesions the intensity of nonphosphorylated neurofilament staining was reduced. Neuritic ovoids were abundant within the cortical lesions. By three-dimensional reconstruction it was found that most of these were connected to only one neuritic process, and thus represented terminal swellings. A few had two neuritic connections, thus representing an en passant dilatation. For most swellings it could not be determined whether it belonged to an axon or a dendrite, as both contain nonphosphorylated neurofilament. Confocal double-labeling microscopy showed that microglia extended processes to and ensheathed neuritic elements and neuronal cell bodies in cortical lesions. Neuronal apoptosis in cortical lesions was studied by TUNEL and neurofilament immunocytochemistry. TUNEL-positive apoptotic neurons were detected in 10 of 22 cortical lesions. The density of apoptotic neurons per cortical lesion area was determined by morphometric analysis to be 1.4 cells per 100 mm^2, vs 0.01 cell per 100 mm^2 in nondemyelinated adjacent cortex. This difference was statistically significant ($p<0.05$). Most apoptotic neurons were large and pyramidal, located in cortical layers 3 and 5.

The extent of neuronal loss in the thalamus in MS was studied by Cifelli et al. in autopsy specimens from 10 MS patients and 10 controls [21]. The density of neurons in the medial dorsal nucleus of the thalamus was reduced by 22%, and the medial dorsal volume and whole thalamic volume were reduced by 21% and 22%, respectively. From these data a 35% total reduction in number of neurons relative to controls was estimated. This corresponded to an estimate of 30% effective neuronal volume loss on the basis of magnetic resonance spectroscopy. The possible presence of thalamic grey matter lesions was not studied, so it is unknown whether this neuronal loss was associated with local GM lesions or was a result of adjacent or distant inflammation, demyelination, and axonal loss. Evangelou et al. found a correlation between axonal loss in optic nerves and measures of neuronal pathology in the parvocellular layer of the lateral geniculate nucleus, suggesting that grey matter neuronal damage can occur as a result of white matter axonal damage [22]. Neuronal pathology in cortical lesions may include synaptic loss, as a 26% decrease in synaptophysin immunoreactivity has been detected in the grey matter part of type 1 lesions, compared with nondemyelinated adjacent cortex [23].

Inflammation

We recently studied the extent of inflammation in grey matter MS lesions in the brains of 10 MS patients [6]. Tissue sections were double-labeled for myelin basic protein and the lymphocyte markers CD3, CD4, CD8, CD45RO, and CD20, and for MHC class II. As described previously [4], we found that MHC class II-positive cells on the border of and within grey matter lesions had the pathology of activated microglia, while in the white matter lesions MHC class II-positive cells were phagocytic macrophages (Fig. 3). Much fewer MHC class II-positive cells were found within grey matter MS lesions than in white matter lesions; this was evident in the combined white matter/grey matter lesions, where white matter phagocytic macrophage infiltration would extend only to the grey matter border (Fig. 3). The highest density of CD3-positive T cells was found in MS white matter lesions. Fewer T cells were detected in cortical lesions that extended through both white and grey matter. The smallest number of T cells was detected in intracortical demyelinated lesions, which had a density of T cells equal to the lymphocyte density in nondemyelinated cerebral cortex within the same tissue block, or cerebral cortex in control brains.

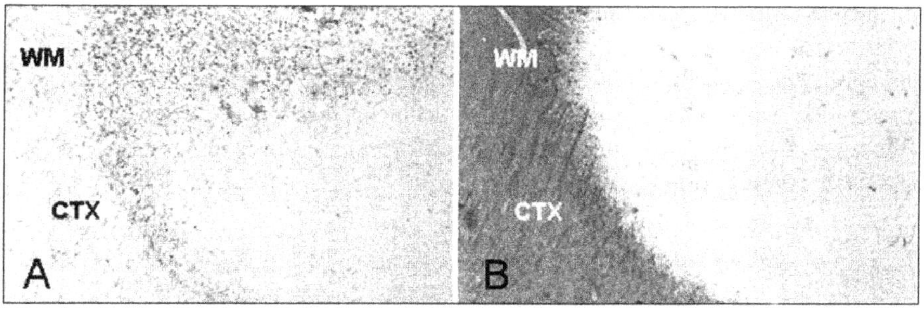

Fig. 3 A-B. Paraffin sections from MS brain immunostained with anti-MHC class II antibody (A), and anti-proteolipid protein (PLP) antibody (B). A combined white matter/grey matter lesion is delineated as an area of loss of PLP staining (B). Abundant infiltration of lipid macrophages is detected in the white matter part of the MS lesion, but not in the cortical part of the lesion (A). Activated microglia are detected at the lesion edge in the cortical part of the lesion (type 1 cortical lesion). *WM*, white matter; *CTX*, cerebral cortex

A similar distribution was found using the CD4, CD8, and CD45RO markers, while CD20-positive B cells were scarce in all specimens examined. Areas of intracortical demyelination in chronic MS were thus not associated with lymphocyte infiltration, or an altered distribution of lymphocyte subsets, when compared with control areas in MS and control patients. This finding indicates that the eventual presence of lymphocyte infiltration in MS lesions is dependent on lesion location.

It is known that there is meningeal lymphocyte infiltration in MS; these infiltrates might secrete substances detrimental to myelin into CSF and adjacent brain tissue. In a pilot study of meningeal inflammation in MS, tissue blocks that contained leptomeningeal tissue from nine control patients and nine MS patients were selected from a large autopsy series [24]. Tissue sections were immunohistochemically stained with anti-CD45, CD3, CD20, and CD117 antibodies for leukocytes, T cells, B cells, and mast cells, respectively. The densities of CD45-, CD3-, and CD20-positive cells were significantly increased in meninges in MS brain. There was a nonsignificant trend toward a higher extent of leukocyte infiltration over cortical lesions. The density of leukocytes in MS was higher in meninges than within white matter lesions. There was thus significant meningeal leukocyte infiltration with T cells, monocytes, and B cells in MS, but the relationship with lesions was not clear.

Conclusions

There is a paucity of studies on the histopathology of the grey matter in MS, with very little information on normal-appearing grey matter. The sensitivity of MRI for grey matter MS lesions appears to be low; normal-appearing grey matter on MRI is thus made up of both lesional and nonlesional tissue. Grey matter demyelination has been described in several studies as a process of selective myelin loss, with much less associated inflammation and disruption of the cytoarchitecture than in white matter. Nevertheless, neuronal and axonal pathology also occurs within cortical lesion areas.

References

1. Prineas JW, McDonald WI, Franklin RJM (2002) Demyelinating diseases In: Graham DI, Lantos PL (eds) Greenfield's neuropathology. Arnold, London, pp 471-550
2. Brownell BHJT (1962) The distribution of plaques in the cerebrum in multiple sclerosis. J Neurol Neurosurg Psychiatry 25:315-321
3. Kidd D, Barkhof F, McConnell R et al (1999) Cortical lesions in multiple sclerosis. Brain 122(Pt 1):17-26
4. Peterson JW, Bö L, Mörk SJ et al (2001) Transected neurites, apoptotic neurons, and reduced inflammation in cortical multiple sclerosis lesions. Ann Neurol 50:389-400
5. Bö L, Vedeler CA, Nyland HI et al (2003) Subpial demyelination in the cerebral cortex of multiple sclerosis patients. J Neuropathol Exp Neurol 62:723-732
6. Bö L, Vedeler CA, Nyland H et al (2003) Intracortical multiple sclerosis lesions are not associated with increased lymphocyte infiltration. Mult Scler 9:323-331
7. Geurts JJG, Bö L, Castelijns JA et al (2004) Cortical lesions in multiple sclerosis: a combined post mortem MRI and histopathology study. AJNR Am J Neuroradiol (in press)
8. Sander M (1898) Hirnrindenbefunde bei multipler Sklerose. Monatschr Psychiatr Neurol IV:427-436
9. Dinkler (1904) Zur Kasuistik der multiplen Herdsklerose des Gehirns und Rückenmarks. Dtsch Zeitschr Nervenheilkd 26:233-247
10. Schob F (1907) Ein Beitrag zur patologischen Anatomie der multiplen Sklerose. Monatschr Psychiatr Neurol 22:62-87
11. Dawson JW (1916) The Histology Of Disseminated Sclerosis. Trans R Soc Edin L:517-774
12. Newcombe J, Hawkins CP, Henderson CL et al (1991) Histopathology of multiple sclerosis lesions detected by magnetic resonance imaging in unfixed postmortem central nervous system tissue. Brain 114:1013-1023
13. Thompson AJ, Kermode AG, Moseley IF et al (1993) Seizures due to multiple sclerosis: seven patients with MRI correlations. J Neurol Neurosurg Psychiatry 56:1317-1320
14. Moriarty DM, Blackshaw AJ, Talbot PR et al (1999) Memory dysfunction in multiple sclerosis corresponds to juxtacortical lesion load on fast fluid-attenuated inversion-recovery MR images. AJNR Am J Neuroradiol 20:1956-1962
15. Lazeron RH, Langdon DW, Filippi M et al (2000) Neuropsychological impairment in multiple sclerosis patients: the role of (juxta)cortical lesion on FLAIR. Mult Scler 6:280-285
16. Rovaris M, Filippi M, Minicucci L et al (2000) Cortical/subcortical disease burden and cognitive impairment in patients with multiple sclerosis. AJNR Am J Neuroradiol 21:402-408
17. Feinstein A, Roy P, Lobaugh N et al (2004) Structural brain abnormalities in multiple sclerosis patients with major depression. Neurology 62:586-590
18. Itoyama Y, Sternberger NH, Webster HD et al (1980) Immuno-cytochemical observations on the distribution of myelin-associated glycoprotein and myelin basic-protein in multiple-sclerosis lesions. Ann Neurol 7:167-177

19. Lumsden CE (1970) The neuropathology of multiple sclerosis. In: Vinken PJ, Bruyn GW (eds) Handbook of clinical neurology. Multiple sclerosis and other demyelinating diseases. Amsterdam, North Holland, pp 217-309
20. Hellwig B (1993) How the myelin picture of the human cerebral cortex can be computed from cytoarchitectural data. A bridge between von Economo and Vogt. J Hirnforsch 34:387-402
21. Cifelli A, Arridge M, Jezzard P et al (2002) Thalamic neurodegeneration in multiple sclerosis. Ann Neurol 52:650-653
22. Evangelou N, Konz D, Esiri MM et al (2001) Size-selective neuronal changes in the anterior optic pathways suggest a differential susceptibility to injury in multiple sclerosis. Brain 124:1813-1820
23. Wegner C, Esiri MM, Palace J, Matthews PM (2003) Synaptic loss in cortical lesions of multiple sclerosis. Mult Scler 9:P612
24. Bö L, van den Berg H, van der Valk P (2003) Meningeal inflammation, a cause of demyelination in multiple sclerosis? J Pathol 201:8A-8A

Chapter 10

Imaging Cerebral Grey Matter Volume in Multiple Sclerosis

N. De Stefano

Introduction

Axonal and neuronal pathology have recently been increasingly regaining attention in multiple sclerosis (MS). There has been a shift in focus from considering functional impairment as primarily resulting from changes in the electrical conduction properties of axons after demyelination, towards an appreciation of the apparently primary role of neurodegeneration in the pathogenesis of this disease. Brain atrophy, which constantly occurs and progressively increases in MS patients, has greatly contributed to the development of this concept. As an expression of general tissue loss, brain atrophy is generally considered a global marker of adverse disease outcome. This seems to include, even in a primarily demyelinating disease such as MS, grey matter (GM) tissue abnormality. Accordingly, selective pathology in the cerebral GM has been shown in recent post-mortem [1-3] and in vivo [4-9] MS studies suggesting that neocortical pathology is more relevant in MS than previously thought.

Diffuse Brain Atrophy in MS

Cerebral atrophy occurs in most neurodegenerative disorders with a mechanism that is mostly driven by neuronal and axonal loss [10, 11]. However, the pathological correlates of brain atrophy in MS are likely to be more complex. Demyelination and inflammation are additional major pathological hallmarks of MS, and, as a consequence, loss of brain tissues such as myelin and glial cells might contribute significantly to the total loss of tissue volume occurring in MS brains [12, 13]. Thus, brain atrophy should be considered in this disease as an expression of a generalized process that involves various brain tissue components.

The ability to measure brain volumes from conventional magnetic resonance (MR) images with methods that can be easily implemented at any MR centre has increased the interest in brain atrophy as an index for accurate assessment and monitoring of the pathological evolution of MS. Several recent studies have shown that cerebral atrophy can be accurately determined from conventional T_1-weighted (T_1-W) MR images with the aid of specific methods allowing computed measurements of total brain volume. Using these methods, significant atrophy has been recently reported in the brains of MS patients in both cross-sectional and longitudinal studies [14-21]. In particular, diffuse brain volume loss has been found in MS patients with mild disability [16], and significantly increased rates of ventricular enlargement have been reported both in early-stage MS patients [18] and patients with clinically isolated syndromes who later developed MS [20].

Methods of Brain Volume Measurement

Given the increasing interest in assessing and monitoring brain atrophy in MS, several manual, semi-manual, and fully automatic approaches to measuring brain volume changes have been developed over the last few years [13]. *Manual measures* of brain volume loss rely upon linear measures of the width of the brain, the corpus callosum, and the third and lateral ventricles [13]. Measurements of these regions have the advantages of being relatively simple and performed on non-digitized data. However, these methods are poorly reproducible even in very experienced hands. *Semi-automatic methods* can measure brain volume changes more directly. In the method described by Loseff et al. [14], for example, a large central volume of brain is defined based on anatomical criteria, the brain is separated from the skull in each slice of the volume, and the aggregate is recorded at each time point. This method appears accurate, gives reproducible results, and has been extensively used in clinical studies. However, semi-automatic methods have the disadvantage of the bias potentially coming from user interventions such as, for example, the selection of brain slices. *Fully automatic* approaches [16, 21-23] do not suffer from this potential bias and have the advantage of measuring the total brain volume. This can be done, as in the brain parenchymal fraction approach [16], by computing the volume of the brain from measurements of the difference in volumes inside a mesh over the exterior surface of the brain and inside the ventricles. This method seems to be highly accurate and produces highly reproducible results. However, a more precise measurement can be probably obtained when serial scans from an individual are accurately registered and the cerebral volume changes are derived directly [22].

The SIENA (Structural Image Evaluation using Normalization, of Atrophy) method [21] is an increasingly used fully automatic method for directly assessing brain volume changes. SIENA decreases variance in measurements of volume change by estimating directly the local shifts in the brain edges rather than average changes in volumes across the entire brain. In the SIENA longitudinal method, the external surface of the skull is used as an invariant constraint on serial images, which is usually clearly visible on T_1-W images. The brain is segmented from non-brain using 3D triangulated mesh modelling to the brain surface, a procedure that balances local and global constraints and uses a local threshold and smoothness factor to reliably detect the brain surface. Once the brain surface is found on one scan, the programme then finds surface point positions to sub-voxel accuracy between scans at two different time points using correlation of normal vectors. This is then converted into percentage brain volume changes. The precision and accuracy of percentage brain volume change is around 0.2%. Since each brain is matched against itself at another time point, it potentially has higher precision than methods that measure total brain volume change. The SIENA method has also been developed to compare single time-point measures (SIENAX) [24], using the skull-based registration process to normalize for head size, and tissue segmentation (expectation-maximization iteration of bias field correction and Markhov random field-Bayesian segmentation) to find brain volume. This method gives a test-retest reproducibility of brain volume measures of about 1%. Both longitudinal and cross-sectional methods can be extended to include selective measures of specific brain compartments by using standard-space masks. Thus, regional atrophy variations such as, for example, total GM changes or selective neocortical volume decreases can be measured.

Grey Matter Atrophy in MS

The relative contributions of the different tissue compartments to brain atrophy and, in particular, the importance of neocortical pathology in this process can be investigated by selectively assessing GM volumes in MS patients. Thus, a number of computational methods for cross-sectional measurements of regional brain volumes have been used successfully in several recent clinical studies to measure GM volume in a range of patients with different forms of MS [6, 7, 23, 25]. Using these methods, many studies have consistently demonstrated that GM atrophy is prominent in MS from the earliest disease stages [6, 7, 23]. Neocortical volume decreases were found, for example [7], in both relapsing-remitting (RR) and primary progressive (PP) MS patients, even when patients were grouped for short disease duration (<5 years) or for low cerebral lesion load [<5 ml of T_2-weighted (T_2-W) lesions], suggesting that neocortical pathology not only occurs at the earliest stages of MS, but also appears to be significant even with minimal white matter lesion accumulation.

The concept that, in a demyelinating disorder such as MS, a cortical pathology can not only be prominent from early disease stages, but can be at least partially independent of white matter lesion genesis is new and important. Indeed, this is strongly suggested by all GM volumetric MR studies so far reported [6, 7, 23, 25]. In these studies, the modest relationship found between T_2-W lesion volume and GM volume measures in RRMS patients (which explained, in some cases, no more than the 25% of the variance in the neocortical measure [7]) and the complete absence of this relationship in PPMS patients [7] lend support to the hypothesis that GM atrophy is not necessarily dependent on cerebral white matter changes. In addition, recently, Sailer and co-workers [26], by using a novel approach to image analysis that allows highly precise measurements of thickness all across the cortex, demonstrated about a 30% decrease in cortical thickness in MS patients relative to age-matched healthy controls. In their elegant work, they also showed that cortical thinning can be predominant in the superior temporal gyrus and the superior and middle frontal gyri in MS patients with short disease course, low disability, and low white matter lesions. Thus, these results provide evidence that there are specific brain GM regions that can be earlier and more deeply involved than others in the pathological process and provide new evidence of the high relevance of a primary cortical pathology from the earliest stages of MS.

These conclusions rely on accurate segmentation of grey and white matter in the MR images. A methodological concern is that apparent decreases in GM volumes might be related to the presence of occult neocortical inflammatory lesions. Such lesions can be seen consistently in post-mortem studies [1, 2], but are rarely detected on MRI using conventional sequences [27, 28]. Thus, subtle changes in MR signal intensity due to neocortical lesions undetectable on MR could affect segmentation between the cortex and cerebrospinal fluid such that the cortex appears to decrease in volume. However, as the presence of significant GM volume decreases was found in several studies in patients with minimal T_2-W white matter lesion accumulation [6, 7, 26], it is very unlikely that the detected decrease in GM volumes could be due primarily to a neocortical lesion burden. As mentioned before, MR data more likely suggest that, while a significant portion of neuroaxonal damage is dependent on focal white matter changes, the GM pathology occurring in MS can be due also to mechanisms independent of lesion genesis.

Clinical Relevance of GM Atrophy in MS

Clinical-pathological correlations have been investigated intensively in MS using different MR techniques. However, the results have often been disappointing. This is undoubtedly due to more than one factor [29, 30], but a contributing element may have been the almost exclusive focus of previous studies on pathological changes in the white matter [2, 30]. Focal white matter lesions do not lead to disability progression in a simple way. A specific illustrative example of this comes from the PP form of MS, which is usually characterized by high disability with low white matter lesion load. Another example is seen in the cognitive dysfunction which is present in about 40-60% of MS patients and cannot be fully explained with white matter lesions alone [31, 32].

The changes occurring in the GM can probably better elucidate both these points. The results of GM volumetric studies showed that, whereas in RRMS patients the amount of GM atrophy seems to correlate moderately with T_2-W brain lesions and (somewhat more weakly) with disease duration, GM volume loss does not seem to contribute significantly to the extent of clinical disability in this form of the disease [6, 7, 23, 25]. In contrast, a very close relationship between GM volume loss and clinical disability can be found in PPMS patients, but they do not show significant correlations between measures of clinical disability and those of T_2-W lesion volume or disease duration [7]. Thus, MR data support the hypothesis of potential clinical-pathological differences between the two forms of the disease [33-36] and suggest that in the PP more than in the RR form of MS, neocortical atrophy might be due to a pathological process that is mostly dominated by neurodegeneration and that, regardless of the mechanisms, seems to be very relevant to clinical disability.

As mentioned above, cognitive impairment can be demonstrated in a great number of MS patients [31], even including a proportion of those with very early-stage disease [32, 37]. This has been considered generally to be strictly dependent on white matter changes and, possibly, subcortical pathology [38-40]. However, although increasing cognitive impairment may sometimes proceed in parallel with increasing T2-W MR lesion load, the magnitude of the correlation between neuropsychological scores and T2-W lesions has been generally modest [38, 39, 41]. As MRI-visible T2-W lesions represent only part of the MS pathology, and brain tissue apparently normal on conventional MR seems to have a great pathological relevance in the disease [42], pathology occurring in normal-appearing brain tissue may be relevant to understanding the process underlying cognitive dysfunction in MS [41]. In agreement with this, cognitive impairment has been associated in many MR studies with measures of cerebral atrophy, and the importance of decreasing brain volumes, rather than increasing lesion load, to MS-related cognitive impairment has been demonstrated even in early RRMS patients [43]. More recently, the specific contribution of the neocortical pathology to MS-related cognitive impairment has been assessed by selectively measuring neocortical volumes in RRMS patients with mild cognitive impairment [44]. In this study, after grouping patients with cognitive impairment and patients with preserved cognition according to their performance on neuropsychological tests, significant decreases in neocortical volume were exclusively found in the first group. In addition, only cognitively impaired MS patients showed a close relationship between measures of neocortical atrophy and both global measures of the degree of cognitive impairment and selective measures of cognitive dysfunction such as defects in verbal and spatial memory, sustained attention and concentration, and verbal fluency. This suggests that the measure of cortical volume may be a sensitive indicator of even mild cognitive impairment and, most of all, implies that neocortical pathology is relevant to cognitive impairment in MS.

Other MR Indicators of GM Pathology in MS

As mentioned before, conventional MR imaging is relatively insensitive to GM pathology. However, as more sensitive MR techniques have come into use, the contribution of GM to the total brain pathology in MS has shown to be substantial. In this context, magnetization transfer imaging [9, 45], diffusion tensor MRI

[5, 46], and MR spectroscopy [3, 4, 8, 47, 48] have been increasingly used in addition to MR measures of GM atrophy to define MS GM pathology not visible on conventional MRI scans. Measurements of proton MR spectroscopy, for example, have shown significant decreases in *N*-acetylaspartate (NAA) in the neocortex of MS patients, consistent with neuronal or axonal injury [3, 4, 8, 47, 48]. In one of these studies, Cifelli and co-workers [3] demonstrated neurodegeneration in the thalamus of secondary progressive MS patients by using MR spectroscopy and histopathological methods in parallel. More recently, this work has been extended into RRMS [8]. In both studies, the amount of ex vivo total loss of thalamic neurons was largely comparable to the neurodegeneration defined in vivo by the decrease in relative NAA concentration and in thalamic volume loss.

Together, these non-conventional MR measures add to those of GM atrophy in emphasizing that GM pathology contributes a substantial proportion to the load of disease in MS. The differences between different MR measures in sensitivity to grey and white matter abnormalities emphasize the need for the simultaneous use of multiple MR-based techniques to assess the full range of pathology in this disease.

Mechanisms of GM Changes in MS

While post-mortem and in vivo studies have demonstrated both focal and diffuse GM changes in MS brains, the mechanisms underlying GM pathology are not fully clarified. The most accepted hypothesis is that axonal damage may lead to retrograde neurodegeneration [49]. As the corticospinal tracts and the frontal periventricular white matter are preferential sites for MS white matter lesions [41], white matter pathology in MS may lead to selective retrograde injury to frontal, temporal, and motor areas of the cortex. This could explain, for example, the characteristic pattern of the focal cortical thinning found in the study by Sailer and co-workers mentioned above. The results of other studies [7, 49], however, suggest that retrograde changes from focal white matter lesions cannot satisfactorily explain the full range of findings.

An alternative to the hypothesis that axonal injury might be associated with neuronal dystrophy through anterograde and retrograde changes [50] is the possibility that a primary neuronal loss may underlie some of the diffuse axonal destruction detected in the normal-appearing white matter [51]. Experimental studies suggest that, while a proportion of GM changes may be secondary to white matter inflammation, an independent neurodegenerative process also might be active. Neuroaxonal damage and loss may occur via mechanisms that are independent of those causing demyelination, probably related to the presence of an abnormal glia-axonal interaction even with low or absent inflammation [2, 52]. In agreement with this, recent work has shown neuronal apoptosis in experimental allergic encephalomyelitis [53], and apoptotic neuronal death unrelated to axonal transection has been found in the cortex of MS patients [2]. Moreover, by showing decreases in the neuronal marker NAA in both neocortical [54] and subcortical [3] GM of MS patients and by correlating NAA decreases in GM with histopathological findings on post-mortem GM tissue, other studies support the hypothesis that primary neuronal loss could be substantial in MS brains. Thus, while a proportion of this neocortical pathology may be secondary to white matter inflammation, it is credible that an independent neurodegenerative process might also be active.

Conclusions

Although MS is and should still be considered a disease primarily affecting myelinated axons in white matter tracts, GM also is involved in the pathological process and should be considered as an additional location of MS pathology. The mechanisms of this are still unknown and need to be identified. It is likely, however, that cortical inflammatory pathology leading to myelin loss, axonal transection, and neuronal apoptosis can all lead to cortical atrophy [1, 2, 55].

In this context, MR studies have provided unique information. Widespread loss in GM tissue occurs consistently in MS, begins at early disease stages, and can be found in all forms of the disease. To the extent that this damage is irreversible, it must be associated with irreversible neurological dysfunction. Mechanisms of cortical adaptation may be able to maintain normal function and minimize disability from axon injury in the early stages, but can no longer compensate in the later stages of the disease when a threshold of axonal loss is reached and the compensatory resources of the CNS are exhausted [56, 57].

This model of MS and its progression argues strongly for early therapeutic interventions, regardless of disability status, directed not only against inflammation but also towards neuronal protection. Measures of total and regional brain atrophy appear to be important for evaluating strategies for repair, remyelination, and neuroprotection. Longitudinal studies using quantitative approaches to imaging analysis should be carried out to better clarify both these aspects and the time-dependent nature of GM changes and their progressive importance in MS.

Acknowledgements. The study was supported in part by a grant of the Associazione Italiana Sclerosi Multipla.

References

1. Kidd D, Barkhof F, McConnell R et al (1999) Cortical lesions in multiple sclerosis. Brain 122:17-26
2. Peterson JW, Bö L, Mork S, Chang A, Trapp BD (2001) Transected neurites, apoptotic neurons, and reduced inflammation in cortical multiple sclerosis lesions. Ann Neurol 50:389-400
3. Cifelli A, Arridge M, Jezzard P et al (2002) Thalamic neurodegeneration in multiple sclerosis. Ann Neurol 52:650-653

4. Sharma R, Narayana PA, Wolinsky JS (2001) Grey matter abnormalities in multiple sclerosis: proton magnetic resonance spectroscopic imaging. Mult Scler 7:221-226
5. Rovaris M, Bozzali M, Iannucci G et al (2002) Assessment of normal-appearing white and grey matter in patients with primary progressive multiple sclerosis: a diffusion-tensor magnetic resonance imaging study. Arch Neurol 59:1406-1412
6. Chard DT, Griffin CM, Parker GJ et al (2002) Brain atrophy in clinically early relapsing-remitting multiple sclerosis. Brain 125:327-337
7. De Stefano N, Matthews PM, Filippi M et al (2003) Evidence of early cortical atrophy in MS: relevance to white matter changes and disability. Neurology 60:1157-1162
8. Wylezinska M, Cifelli A, Jezzard P et al (2003) Thalamic neurodegeneration in relapsing-remitting multiple sclerosis. Neurology 60:1949-1954
9. Cercignani M, Bozzali M, Iannucci G et al (2001) Magnetisation transfer ratio and mean diffusivity of normal appearing white and grey matter from patients with multiple sclerosis. J Neurol Neurosurg Psychiatry 70:311-317
10. Fox NC, Crum WR, Scahill RI et al (2001) Imaging of onset and progression of Alzheimer's disease with voxel-compression mapping of serial magnetic resonance images. Lancet 358:201-205
11. O'Brien JT, Paling S, Barber R et al (2001) Progressive brain atrophy on serial MRI in dementia with Lewy bodies, AD, and vascular dementia. Neurology 56:1386-1388
12. De Stefano N, Iannucci G, Sormani MP et al (2002) MR correlates of cerebral atrophy in patients with multiple sclerosis. J Neurol 249:1072-1077
13. Miller DH, Barkhof F, Frank JA et al (2002) Measurement of atrophy in multiple sclerosis: pathological basis, methodological aspects and clinical relevance. Brain 125:1676-1695
14. Losseff NA, Wang L, Lai HM et al (1996) Progressive cerebral atrophy in multiple sclerosis. A serial MRI study. Brain 119:2009-2019
15. Simon JH, Jacobs LD, Campion MK et al (1999) A longitudinal study of brain atrophy in relapsing multiple sclerosis. The Multiple Sclerosis Collaborative Research Group (MSCRG). Neurology 53:139-148
16. Rudick RA, Fisher E, Lee JC et al (1999) Use of the brain parenchymal fraction to measure whole brain atrophy in relapsing-remitting MS. Multiple Sclerosis Collaborative Research Group. Neurology 53:1698-1704
17. Liu C, Edwards S, Gong Q et al (1999) Three dimensional MRI estimates of brain and spinal cord atrophy in multiple sclerosis. J Neurol Neurosurg Psychiatry 66:323-330
18. Luks TL, Goodkin DE, Nelson SJ et al (2000) A longitudinal study of ventricular volume in early relapsing-remitting multiple sclerosis. Mult Scler 6:332-337
19. Fox NC, Jenkins R, Leary SM et al (2000) Progressive cerebral atrophy in MS: a serial study using registered, volumetric MRI. Neurology 54:807-812
20. Brex PA, Jenkins R, Fox NC et al (2000) Detection of ventricular enlargement in patients at the earliest clinical stage of MS. Neurology 54:1689-1691
21. Smith SM, De Stefano N, Jenkinson M, Matthews PM (2001) Normalized accurate measurement of longitudinal brain change. J Comput Assist Tomogr 25:466-475
22. Freeborough PA, Fox NC (1997) The boundary shift integral: an accurate and robust measure of cerebral volume changes from registered repeat MRI. IEEE Trans Med Imaging 16:623-629
23. Quarantelli M, Ciarmiello A, Morra VB et al (2003) Brain tissue volume changes in relapsing-remitting multiple sclerosis: correlation with lesion load. Neuroimage 18:360-366
24. Smith SM, Zhang Y, Jenkinson M et al (2002) Accurate, robust and automated longitudinal and cross-sectional brain change analysis. Neuroimage 17:479-489
25. Ge Y, Grossman RI, Udupa JK et al (2001) Brain atrophy in relapsing-remitting multiple sclerosis: fractional volumetric analysis of grey matter and white matter. Radiology 220:606-610

26. Sailer M, Fischl B, Salat D et al (2003) Focal thinning of the cerebral cortex in multiple sclerosis. Brain 126:1734-1744
27. Bakshi R, Dmochowski J, Shaikh ZA, Jacobs L (2001) Grey matter T2 hypointensity is related to plaques and atrophy in the brains of multiple sclerosis patients. J Neurol Sci 185:19-26
28. Bakshi R, Benedict RH, Bermel RA et al (2002) T2 hypointensity in the deep grey matter of patients with multiple sclerosis: a quantitative magnetic resonance imaging study. Arch Neurol 59:62-68
29. McDonald WI (1994) Rachelle Fishman-Matthew Moore Lecture. The pathological and clinical dynamics of multiple sclerosis. [Review.] J Neuropathol Exp Neurol 53:338-343
30. Trapp BD, Ransohoff RM, Fisher E, Rudick RA (1999) Neurodegeneration in multiple sclerosis: relationship to neurological disability. Neuroscientist 5:48-57
31. Rao SM, Leo GJ, Bernardin L, Unverzagt F (1991) Cognitive dysfunction in multiple sclerosis. I. Frequency, patterns, and prediction. Neurology 41:685-691
32. Feinstein A, Youl B, Ron M (1992) Acute optic neuritis. A cognitive and magnetic resonance imaging study. Brain 115:1403-1415
33. Thompson AJ, Polman CH, Miller DH et al (1997) Primary progressive multiple sclerosis. Brain 120:1085-1096
34. Bruck W, Lucchinetti C, Lassmann H (2002) The pathology of primary progressive multiple sclerosis. Mult Scler 8:93-97
35. Revesz T, Kidd D, Thompson AJ, Barnard RO, McDonald WI (1994) A comparison of the pathology of primary and secondary progressive multiple sclerosis. Brain 117:759-765
36. Rovaris M, Bozzali M, Santuccio G et al (2001) In vivo assessment of the brain and cervical cord pathology of patients with primary progressive multiple sclerosis. Brain 124:2540-2549
37. Amato MP, Ponziani G, Pracucci G et al (1995) Cognitive impairment in early-onset multiple sclerosis. Pattern, predictors, and impact on everyday life in a 4-year follow-up. Arch Neurol 52:168-172
38. Rao SM, Leo GJ, Haughton VM et al (1989) Correlation of magnetic resonance imaging with neuropsychological testing in multiple sclerosis. Neurology 39:161-166
39. Rovaris M, Filippi M, Falautano M et al (1998) Relation between MR abnormalities and patterns of cognitive impairment in multiple sclerosis. Neurology 50:1601-1608
40. Lazeron RH, Langdon DW, Filippi M et al (2000) Neuropsychological impairment in multiple sclerosis patients: the role of (juxta)cortical lesion on FLAIR. Mult Scler 6:280-285.
41. Filippi M, Tortorella C, Rovaris M et al (2000) Changes in the normal appearing brain tissue and cognitive impairment in multiple sclerosis. J Neurol Neurosurg Psychiatry 68:157-161
42. Trapp BD, Bö L, Mork S, Chang A (1999) Pathogenesis of tissue injury in MS lesions. J Neuroimmunol 98:49-56
43. Rao SM, Bernardin L, Leo GJ et al (1989) Cerebral disconnection in multiple sclerosis. Relationship to atrophy of the corpus callosum. Arch Neurol 46:918-920
44. Amato MP, Bartolozzi ML, Zipoli V et al (2004) Neocortical volume decrease in relapsing-remitting ms patients with mild cognitive impairment. Neurology (in press)
45. Ge Y, Grossman RI, Udupa JK et al (2001) Magnetization transfer ratio histogram analysis of grey matter in relapsing-remitting multiple sclerosis. AJNR Am J Neuroradiol 22:470-475
46. Bozzali M, Cercignani M, Sormani MP et al (2002) Quantification of brain grey matter damage in different MS phenotypes by use of diffusion tensor MR imaging. AJNR Am J Neuroradiol 23:985-988

47. Kapeller P, McLean MA, Griffin CM et al (2001) Preliminary evidence for neuronal damage in cortical grey matter and normal appearing white matter in short duration relapsing-remitting multiple sclerosis: a quantitative MR spectroscopic imaging study. J Neurol 248:131-138
48. Sarchielli P, Presciutti O, Tarducci R et al (2002) Localized (1)H magnetic resonance spectroscopy in mainly cortical grey matter of patients with multiple sclerosis. J Neurol 249:902-910
49. Evangelou N, Konz D, Esiri MM et al (2001) Size-selective neuronal changes in the anterior optic pathways suggest a differential susceptibility to injury in multiple sclerosis. Brain 124:1813-1820
50. Bjartmar C, Trapp BD (2001) Axonal and neuronal degeneration in multiple sclerosis: mechanisms and functional consequences. Curr Opin Neurol 14:271-278
51. Evangelou N, Esiri MM, Smith S, Palace J, Matthews PM (2000) Quantitative pathological evidence for axonal loss in normal appearing white matter in multiple sclerosis. Ann Neurol 47:391-395
52. Garbern JY, Yool DA, Moore GJ et al (2002) Patients lacking the major CNS myelin protein, proteolipid protein 1, develop length-dependent axonal degeneration in the absence of demyelination and inflammation. Brain 125:551-561
53. Meyer R, Weissert R, Diem R et al (2001) Acute neuronal apoptosis in a rat model of multiple sclerosis. J Neurosci 21:6214-6220
54. Kapeller P, McLean MA, Griffin CM et al (2001) Preliminary evidence for neuronal damage in cortical grey matter and normal appearing white matter in short duration relapsing-remitting multiple sclerosis: a quantitative MR spectroscopic imaging study. J Neurol 248:131-138
55. Lumsden CE (1970) The neuropathology of multiple sclerosis. In: Vinken PJ, Bruyn GW (eds) Handbook of clinical neurology. North Holland and American Elsevier, Amsterdam and New York, pp 296-298
56. Rocca MA, Falini A, Colombo B et al (2002) Adaptive functional changes in the cerebral cortex of patients with nondisabling multiple sclerosis correlate with the extent of brain structural damage. Ann Neurol 51:330-339
57. Cifelli A, Matthews PM (2002) Cerebral plasticity in multiple sclerosis: insights from fMRI. Mult Scler 8:193-199

Chapter 11

The Grey Matter Component of MS Pathology: Magnetization Transfer and Diffusion-Weighted Imaging

M.A. Rocca, M. Filippi

Introduction

The classical view of multiple sclerosis (MS) as a chronic inflammatory disease affecting the white matter (WM) of the central nervous system (CNS) has been recently challenged by pathological studies and by the extensive application of modern magnetic resonance imaging (MRI)-based techniques, including magnetization transfer (MT) MRI and diffusion-weighted (DW) MRI. These techniques have overcome some of the limitations of conventional MRI, such as its poor specificity to the heterogeneous pathological substrates of the disease, and have demonstrated that: (1) axonal pathology in macroscopic brain lesions and in normal-appearing brain tissue is an important feature of MS from its earliest phase; (2) grey matter (GM) is not spared by the pathological process in MS; and (3) brain plasticity might contribute to clinical recovery and the maintenance of a normal level of function in the presence of MS-related irreversible tissue loss.

In this chapter, we summarize the main results obtained by the application of MT and DW MRI to the quantification of GM pathology in MS, highlighting how they are changing our understanding of MS, which is now viewed as a CNS condition affecting both WM and GM and which causes irreversible clinical disability mainly through axonal/neuronal damage.

Pathological Abnormalities in the Grey Matter

Brownell and Hughes were the first to quantify GM involvement in MS patients [1]. In a study of 32 cases of MS, these authors identified 1594 cerebral plaques. Twenty-six percent of these plaques involved the GM (17% were at the junction of the cortex and the WM, 5% were restricted to the cortex, and 4% were in the central GM). The frequency of GM involvement in MS was underlined in a subsequent study by Lumsden [2], who detected variable numbers of MS lesions within the cerebral cortex of 93% of 60 cases studied. More recently, Kidd et al. [3] detected 478 GM lesions (76% with involvement of the subcortical WM, 24% located exclusively within the cortex) at postmortem examination of 12 cases of MS. Peterson et al. [4] identified 112 GM lesions in 50 cases of MS: 34% of these lesions incorporated both the WM and the cortex (type I), 16% were located entirely within the cortex (type II), and the remaining 50% extended from the pial surface into the cortex (type III). More recently, an additional pattern of cortical involvement (type IV), characterized by lesion extension though the whole width of the cortex, without reaching the subcortical WM, has been described [5]. Compared to WM lesions, GM lesions have different pathological characteristics: they have fewer lymphocytes, microglia, and perivascular cuffs; in other words, these lesions tend to have less inflammatory infiltrate than those located in the WM, thus appearing hypocellular [3-5].

Conventional MRI Studies

GM lesions are usually missed on conventional T2-weighted images because they are small [3] and have longer relaxation times than normal WM, which results in poor contrast resolution between them and surrounding normal GM; and also, in the case of cortical lesions, because of partial volume effects with cerebrospinal fluid (CSF).

Among the strategies applied to increase GM lesion detection, the most promising seem to be the use of fast fluid-attenuated inversion recovery (fast-FLAIR) sequences and the acquisition of T_1-weighted sequences after the administration of gadolinium (Gd). Due to CSF signal suppression, fast-FLAIR sequences allow a greater number of cortical and juxtacortical lesions to be detected than do T_2-weighted sequences [3, 6], while the use of Gd greatly increases the number of new cortical lesions seen (up to 140% in comparison to other techniques) [3]. GM involvement in MS patients is not limited to the cortical GM, but also extensively involves the deep GM, as indicated by several studies which found T_2 hypointensity, probably reflecting iron deposition, in deep GM of MS patients [7].

A global and precise quantification of GM damage in MS patients might allow the strength of the correlation between clinical and MRI findings to increase, and might help to explain some MS symptoms such as cognitive impairment and fatigue. However, studies aimed at improving these correlations have given disappointing results. Catalaa et al. [8] found no relationship between GM lesions and cognitive function in 18 patients with relapsing-remitting (RR) MS, while Lazeron et al. [9] found only a moderate correlation (r=0.34) between these two variables.

Modern structural MR-based techniques with increased specificity to the heterogeneous pathological substrates of MS have the potential to overcome the limitations of conventional MRI for detection and quantification of GM abnormalities, and might improve our understanding of how MS evolves.

Basic Principles of MT and DW MRI

MT MRI is based on the interactions between protons in a relatively free environment and those where motion is restricted. Off-resonance irradiation is applied, which saturates the magnetization of the less mobile protons, but this is transferred to the mobile protons, thus reducing the signal intensity from the observable magnetization. Thus, a low MT ratio (MTR) indicates a reduced capacity of the macromolecules in the CNS to exchange magnetization with the surrounding water molecules, reflecting damage to myelin or to the axonal membrane. The most compelling evidence indicating that markedly decreased MTR values correspond to areas where severe and irreversible tissue loss has occurred comes from a postmortem study showing a strong correlation of MTR values from MS lesions and normal-appearing WM (NAWM) with the percentage of residual axons and the degree of demyelination [10].

Diffusion is the microscopic random translational motion of molecules in a fluid system. Water molecular diffusion can be measured in vivo using DW MRI, in terms of an apparent diffusion coefficient (ADC) [11]. Although diffusion is inherently a three-dimensional process, in some tissues with an oriented microstructure, such as brain WM, the molecular mobility is not the same in all directions. This property is called anisotropy, and results in a variation of the measured diffusivity with tissue measurement direction. WM fiber tracts consist of aligned myelinated axons, and therefore hindrance of water diffusion is much greater across than it is along the major axis of axonal fibers. Under these conditions, a full characterization of diffusion can only be found in terms of a tensor, a 3×3 matrix, where the on-diagonal elements represent the diffusion coefficients along the axes of the reference frame, while the off-diagonal elements account for the correlations between molecular displacement along orthogonal directions [12]. From the tensor, it is possible to derive some scalar indices [11]. These include the mean diffusivity (MD) (equal to one-third of the trace of the diffusion tensor), which is affected by cellular size and integrity, and the fractional anisotropy (FA), which reflects the degree of alignment of cellular structures within fiber tracts, as well as their structural integrity.

Both MT and DW MRI have substantial advantages over conventional MRI in the study of MS [11, 13]. First, they provide quantitative information with increased specificity to the heterogeneous substrates of MS pathology. Secondly, they enable us to quantify the diffuse damage occurring in brain tissues that appear normal on conventional MRI. Thirdly, with the application of histogram analysis, they can provide multiple parameters influenced by both the conventional MRI-visible and "occult" lesion burdens.

MT MRI Studies of Normal-Appearing GM

Using region-of-interest (ROI) analysis, several authors found no abnormalities in the cortical [14-16] and deep [14, 15, 17] normal-appearing GM (NAGM) of MS patients.

The application of histogram analysis has allowed the demonstration in vivo of the widespread MT MRI abnormalities of MS patients' NAGM. Ge et al. [18]

found a reduction of NAGM MTR values in a group of 18 patients with RRMS compared to healthy volunteers. In MS patients, the reduction of NAGM MTR values was strongly related with Expanded Disability Status Scale (EDSS) scores (r=–0.65) and with brain T_2-weighted lesion volumes (r=–0.55). A reduction of NAGM MTR values, moderately correlated to T_2 lesion volumes, has also been found by Cercignani et al., using a different segmentation technique [19]. Interestingly, in this study, a reduction of NAGM MTR values was also found using ROI analysis. The discrepancy between this finding and those of previous studies [14-16] might be related either to the size of the ROIs used (relatively large ROIs have a greater likelihood of being contaminated incidentally by CSF, biasing the measurements) or to the number and location of these ROIs. The correlations reported by these authors between GM MTR histographic changes and T_2 lesion volume [18, 19] indicate that at least part of GM pathology in MS is secondary to retrograde degeneration of fibers traversing WM lesions.

More recently, NAGM abnormalities have also been demonstrated in patients with the progressive phenotypes of the disease [20, 21]. Such changes are more pronounced in patients with secondary progressive (SP) MS than in those with RRMS [20]. In patients with primary progressive (PP) MS, NAGM MTR reduction is correlated with worsening in EDSS scores (r=–0.41) [21].

Cortical/subcortical brain tissue MTR [22], but not basal ganglia MTR [23], was found to differ significantly between MS patients and healthy controls and to correlate strongly with MS cognitive impairment [22]. However, GM MTR histograms were not different between patients with and without fatigue [23].

DW MRI Studies of NAGM

Consistent with pathological [1-5] and MT MRI [18-21] studies, GM involvement in MS has been also demonstrated using DW MRI [19, 24, 25]. After having segmented GM from WM using a threshold based on their different anisotropic characteristics, Cercignani et al. [19] demonstrated that, in comparison to sex- and age-matched healthy volunteers, MS patients have increased MD histogram-derived metrics of brain NAGM. Using the same technique, Bozzali et al. [24] have recently demonstrated that NAGM changes are more pronounced in patients with SPMS and PPMS than in patients with the RR course of the disease, whereas Rovaris et al. [25] showed that NAWM and NAGM pathology is more severe in patients with SPMS than in patients with PPMS. These findings suggest that NAGM pathological abnormalities might yet be an additional factor contributing to the worsening of clinical disability in patients with progressive MS. As previously shown by MT MRI studies [18, 19], in all these DW MRI studies [19, 24, 25] moderate correlations have been found between NAGM MD histogram-derived metrics and brain T_2-weighted lesion loads, indicating that part of GM pathology in MS is secondary to retrograde degeneration of fibers traversing T_2-visible lesions.

The presence of NAGM damage in MS fits well with the frequent demonstration of cognitive impairment in patients with MS. Rovaris et al. [26] found a moderate correlation between the level of cognitive impairment and MD of the NAGM in 34 mildly disabled RRMS patients.

GM abnormalities have also been demonstrated by pathological assessment [27] in the basal ganglia of MS patients. While in a preliminary study of 31 patients with MS, no DWI changes were found in these deep GM structures [17], a more recent study, performed in 82 MS patients, showed increased ADC values in the thalami of MS patients in comparison with those of healthy volunteers [28]. Basal ganglia GM DWI changes are also more pronounced in SPMS than in RRMS patients. This finding of basal ganglia DWI abnormalities suggests that the positron emission tomography [29] and functional MRI [30] changes detected in the basal ganglia of MS patients are likely to be secondary to intrinsic structural changes.

More recently, the feasibility of longitudinal DT MRI assessment has been demonstrated [31]. In a 18-month follow-up study conducted in 26 patients with RRMS, Oreja-Guevara et al. [31] showed that NAGM changes worsen over time in MS. This suggests a progressive accumulation of GM damage already in the RR phase of the disease, which was previously unrecognized and which might be one of the factors responsible for the development of brain atrophy [32] and neuropsychological impairment.

Recent developments in DTI techniques have enabled tracing of large fiber tracts in the human brain [33, 34]. However, the conventional algorithms used to trace WM tracts have limited usefulness in defining pathways near GM, due to uncertainty of fiber direction at this level. Using a probabilistic tractography algorithm, Behrens et al. [35] have recently demonstrated that it is possible to trace connections from the thalamus to the GM of the human cerebral cortex using DTI. The application of this method to the study of MS patients might provide important information about MS brain connectivity.

Conclusions

At present, GM pathology is a well-established feature of MS. Modern MR-based techniques, such as MT and DW MRI, provide quantitative and reproducible measures which allow accurate quantification of GM damage. Future research work should extend the application of these techniques to larger sample of MS patients, in order to improve our ability to monitor the disease and improve the correlation between MRI metrics and disability.

References

1. Brownell B, Hughes JT (1962) The distribution of plaques in the cerebrum in multiple sclerosis. J Neurol Neurosurg Psychiatry 25:315-320

2. Lumsden CE (1970) The neuropathology of multiple sclerosis. In: Vinken PJ, Bruyn GW (eds) Handbook of clinical neurology, vol 9. Amsterdam, North-Holland, pp 217-309
3. Kidd D, Barkhof F, McConnell R, Algra PR, Allen IV, Revesz T (1999) Cortical lesions in multiple sclerosis. Brain 122:17-26
4. Peterson JW, Bö L, Mork S, Chang A, Trapp BD (2001) Transected neurites, apoptotic neurons, and reduced inflammation in cortical multiple sclerosis lesions. Ann Neurol 50:389-400
5. Bo L, Vedeler CA, Nyland H, Trapp BD, Mork SJ (2003) Intracortical multiple sclerosis lesions are not associated with increased lymphocyte infiltration. Mult Scler 9:323-331
6. Bakshi R, Ariyaratana S, Benedict RH, Jacobs L (2001) Fluid-attenuated inversion recovery magnetic resonance imaging detects cortical and juxtacortical multiple sclerosis lesions. Arch Neurol 58:742-748
7. Bakshi R, Benedict RH, Bermel RA et al (2002) T2 hypointensity in the deep grey matter of patients with multiple sclerosis: a quantitative magnetic resonance imaging study. Arch Neurol 59:62-68
8. Catalaa I, Fulton JC, Zhang X et al (1999) MR imaging quantitation of grey matter involvement in multiple sclerosis and its correlation with disability measures and neurocognitive testing. AJNR Am J Neuroradiol 20:1613-1618
9. Lazeron RH, Langdon DW, Filippi M et al (2000) Neuropsychological impairment in multiple sclerosis patients: the role of (juxta)cortical lesion on FLAIR. Mult Scler 6:280-285
10. van Waesberghe JH, Kamphorst W, De Groot CJ et al (1999) Axonal loss in multiple sclerosis lesions: magnetic resonance imaging insights into substrates of disability. Ann Neurol 46:747-754
11. Filippi M, Inglese M (2001) Overview of diffusion-weighted magnetic resonance studies in multiple sclerosis. J Neurol Sci 186:S37-S43
12. Basser PJ, Mattiello J, Le Bihan D (1994) Estimation of the effective self-diffusion tensor from the NMR spin-echo. J Magn Reson B 103:247-254
13. Filippi M, Grossman RI, Comi G (eds) (1999) Magnetization transfer in multiple sclerosis. Neurology 53 [Suppl 3]
14. Pike GB, de Stefano N, Narayanan S et al (1999) Combined magnetization transfer and proton spectroscopic imaging in the assessment of pathologic brain lesions in multiple sclerosis. AJNR Am J Neuroradiol 20:829-837
15. Santos AC, Narayanan S, de Stefano N et al (2002) Magnetization transfer can predict clinical evolution in patients with multiple sclerosis. J Neurol 249:662-668
16. Griffin CM, Chard DT, Parker GJ et al (2002) The relationship between lesion and normal appearing brain tissue abnormalities in early relapsing remitting multiple sclerosis. J Neurol 249:193-199
17. Filippi M, Bozzali M, Comi G (2001) Magnetization transfer and diffusion tensor MR imaging of basal ganglia from patients with multiple sclerosis. J Neurol Sci 183:69-72
18. Ge Y, Grossman RI, Udupa JK et al (2001) Magnetization transfer ratio histogram analysis of grey matter in relapsing-remitting multiple sclerosis. AJNR Am J Neuroradiol 22:470-475
19. Cercignani M, Bozzali M, Iannucci G et al (2001) Magnetisation transfer ratio and mean diffusivity of normal-appearing white and grey matter from patients with multiple sclerosis. J Neurol Neurosurg Psychiatry 70:311-317
20. Ge Y, Grossman RI, Udupa JK et al (2002) Magnetization transfer ratio histogram analysis of normal-appearing grey matter and normal-appearing white matter in multiple sclerosis. J Comput Assist Tomogr 26:62-68
21. Dehmeshki J, Chard DT, Leary SM et al (2003) The normal appearing grey matter in

primary progressive multiple sclerosis: a magnetisation transfer imaging study. J Neurol 250:67-74

22. Rovaris M, Filippi M, Minicucci L et al (2000) Cortical/subcortical disease burden and cognitive impairment in multiple sclerosis. AJNR Am J Neuroradiol 21:402-408
23. Codella M, Rocca MA, Colombo B et al (2002) Cerebral grey matter pathology and fatigue in patients with multiple sclerosis: a preliminary study. J Neurol Sci 194:71-74
24. Bozzali M, Cercignani M, Sormani MP et al (2002) Quantification of brain grey matter damage in different MS phenotypes by use of diffusion tensor MR imaging. AJNR Am J Neuroradiol 23:985-988
25. Rovaris M, Bozzali M, Iannucci G et al (2002) Assessment of normal-appearing white and grey matter in patients with primary progressive multiple sclerosis: a diffusion-tensor magnetic resonance imaging study. Arch Neurol 59:1406-1412
26. Rovaris M, Iannucci G, Falautano M et al (2002) Cognitive dysfunction in patients with mildly disabling relapsing-remitting multiple sclerosis: an exploratory study with diffusion tensor MR imaging. J Neurol Sci 195:103-109
27. Cifelli A, Arridge M, Jezzard P et al (2002) Thalamic neurodegeneration in multiple sclerosis. Ann Neurol 52:650-653
28. Fabiano AJ, Sharma J, Weinstock-Guttman B et al (2003) Thalamic involvement in multiple sclerosis: a diffusion-weighted magnetic resonance imaging study. J Neuroimaging 13:307-314
29. Roelcke U, Kappos L, Lechner-Scott J et al (1997) Reduced glucose metabolism in the frontal cortex and basal ganglia of multiple sclerosis patients with fatigue: a 18F-fluorodeoxyglucose positron emission tomography study. Neurology 48:1566-1571
30. Filippi M, Rocca MA, Colombo B et al (2002) Functional magnetic resonance imaging correlates of fatigue in multiple sclerosis. Neuroimage 15:559-567
31. Oreja-Guevara C, Rovaris M, Caputo D et al (2003) Changes in cortical grey matter in untreated relapsing-remitting MS patients: a follow up study. Neurology 60:A297
32. Miller DH, Barkhof F, Frank JA et al (2002) Measurement of atrophy in multiple sclerosis: pathological basis, methodological aspects and clinical relevance [review]. Brain 125:1676-1695
33. Jones DK, Simmons A, Williams SC, Horsfield MA (1999) Non-invasive assessment of axonal fiber connectivity in the human brain via diffusion tensor MRI. Magn Reson Med 42:37-41
34. Basser PJ, Pajevic S, Pierpaoli C et al (2000) In vivo fiber tractography using DT-MRI data. Magn Reson Med 44:625-632
35. Behrens TE, Johansen-Berg H, Woolrich MW et al (2003) Non-invasive mapping of connections between human thalamus and cortex using diffusion imaging. Nat Neurosci 6:750-757

Chapter 12

MR Spectroscopy of the Normal-Appearing Grey Matter

O. GONEN, M. INGLESE, R.I. GROSSMAN

Multiple sclerosis (MS) has been regarded for over a hundred years as an inflammatory demyelinating disease affecting the white matter (WM) of the central nervous system (CNS) [1]. Only over the past decade has this perception been expanded to accommodate the mounting pathological and MRI evidence of axonal injury in the WM lesions of the brain and cord [2-5]. This damage has been shown to extend well beyond the macroscopic lesions into the so-called normal-appearing WM (NAWM) with varying degrees of severity and extent [6-11].

Although some evidence that grey matter (GM) is not spared has been available for over 30 years [12, 13], only recently have pathology studies shown cortical and subcortical lesions, usually missed by conventional T_2-weighted MR imaging (T2WI), to be relatively frequent at postmortem exams of deceased MS patients [14-18]. Furthermore, new specialized MR techniques, e.g., magnetization transfer imaging (MTI), diffusion tensor imaging (DTI), and proton magnetic resonance spectroscopy (^{1}H-MRS), frequently reveal abnormal physical properties of the MRI-normal-appearing GM (NAGM) as well [16-19].

In vivo ^{1}H-MRS assessment of the amino acid derivative *N*-acetylaspartate (NAA), which is present almost exclusively in neuronal cells [20], has reported declines in both lesions and NAWM [3, 21-23]. Unfortunately, in the GM ^{1}H-MRS encounters several limitations. First, since cortical GM is only 1-4 mm thick, voxels smaller than 1 cm^3 must be used to reduce WM contamination [24]. Due to signal-to-noise and limited examination time considerations, only one to two such single voxels can be examined per session. Second, the voxels must be placed away from the skull to avoid spectral contamination by intense lipid signals from subcutaneous adipose tissue and bone marrow [25]. Consequently, except for the midline and some of the deep GM nuclei, most cortical GM is difficult to access. Third, poor lesion/GM contrast complicates image guidance to MRI-visible pathology. Fourth, the extensive sulcal structure around the cortex necessitates careful image segmentation to quantify the cerebrospinal fluid (CSF) fraction in each voxel. This must be done to verify whether metabolite level decreases are due to tissue pathology or to partial CSF contamination. This technology is not always available even to sites that routinely perform ^{1}H-MRS. Finally, combinations of the above obstacles render serial studies unreliable due to voxel registration uncertainties.

In this chapter we will cover two approaches, each of which is designed to circumvent the difficulties described above. First, under "Global Evidence of Grey Matter Involvement", we will describe a global, whole-brain approach, to obtain a measure of the concentration of NAA from the entire organ. While this approach avoids the lipids contamination, segmentation, and misregistration issues, it does so at the cost of complete loss of localization [25]. The second, localizing approach, described under "Focal Metabolic Evidence of Deep GM Involvement", uses high spatial resolution (<1-cm^3 voxels) in a three-dimensional (3D) ^{1}H-MRS acquisition scheme. This methodology is used to examine the metabolic abnormalities in the thalamus and basal ganglia of relapsing-remitting (RR) MS patients and compares them with age- and sex- matched controls.

Global Evidence of Grey Matter Involvement

Lipid contamination, voxel misregistration, and poor tissue/lesion contrast and CSF segmentation difficulties can be circumvented by the whole-brain NAA (WBNAA) quantification technique [22, 25]. Although its global coverage comes at a cost of all regional information and maximal GM/WM partial volume admixture, a previous comparison of RRMS patients with matched controls showed upwards of 10% WBNAA deficits as a function of age [22].

Since in RRMS, T_2-visible lesions usually account for less than 3% of the brain volume [26], it was concluded that such losses could only be explained by NAWM involvement [22]. The extent of these deficits motivated us to investigate whether the WM pool was large enough to absorb them. Since the brain's WM and GM volume fractions, in healthy adults, are estimated at 30% and 60%, respectively [27] and the NAA concentration difference between them is reported at approximately 30% [28]; WBNAA deficits exceeding 20% may indicate GM involvement in addition to all the MRI lesions and WM occult pathology.

Methods

Subjects

Seventy-one patients (51 women) with clinically definite RRMS were studied [29]. Their mean age was 38 years (range: 25-55 years), the median disease duration from date of confirmed diagnosis was 5 years (range: 0-22 years), and their median Expanded Disability Status Scale (EDSS) score [30] at the time of this study was 2.0 (range: 0.0-6.0). In addition, 41 healthy controls, (27 women), mean age 37 years (range: 23-55 years) underwent the same procedure. All subjects were briefed on the procedure and gave Institutional Review Board-approved written informed consent.

MRI and GM/WM Segmentation

Each patient's brain volume, V_B, was obtained from proton density (PD) and T_2-weighted fast spin-echo MRI ($TR/TE_1/TE_2$=2500/16/80 ms; 192×256 matrix, 220×220 mm^2 field of view, 3 mm slice thickness) in a 1.5-T scanner. Image segmentation, performed with the Udupa et al. 3DVIEWNIX program [31], started by excluding extracranial content and manually setting several intensity points in the CSF, GM, and WM. The software then used fuzzy-connectedness to create over 50 separate WM (without lesions), GM, and CSF masks per study [32], from which any residual extracranial components were excluded manually. The method was verified with better than 99% reproducibility [33].

Patients' T_2 lesion volumes (T2LV) were also calculated with 3DVIEWNIX, which enables their detection and semiautomatic volume calculation [34]. The operator needs only to accept or reject computer-delineated lesions, maintaining the ability to manually edit under- or overrepresentation. The precision and accuracy of this aspect of the software have been validated and reported elsewhere [34, 35].

WBNAA Acquisition and Quantification

Following global shimming, which yielded consistent 15±3 Hz whole-head water linewidths, the amount of NAA in the head, Q_{NAA}, was obtained using a nonlocalizing, nonecho ^{1}H-MRS sequence (TE/TI/TR=0.0/0.97/10 s) [25]. Each acquisition comprised 16 add–subtract cycles and lasted 2.5 min. Five such measurements were repeated back-to-back for a total of 12 min. The resultant spectrum was processed manually offline using custom software written in the IDL programming language (RSI Inc. Boulder, Colo.). A 2880° first-order (linear) phase shift was applied to the data to undo the baseline-roll of the $1\bar{3}3\bar{1}$ water-suppression readout pulse [25], and an 0th order phase correction was applied to get the (water- and lipids-suppressed) absorption spectrum shown in Fig. 1. Once 0/1st order phased, the two points where the 8-12 Hz fwhm NAA peak intersected the broad (probably amino acid) baseline were manually selected and the program computed the resonance area, S, shown in Fig. 1.

Absolute quantification of Q_{NAA} was done against a reference 3-l (three-liter) sphere of 1.5×10^{-2} mole NAA in water. Subject, S_S, and reference, S_R, NAA peak areas were integrated, as shown in Fig. 1, and Q_{NAA} calculated as [25, 36]:

$$Q_{NAA} = 1.5 \times 10^{-2} \cdot \frac{S_S}{S_R} \cdot \left(\frac{P_S^{180°}}{P_R^{180°}}\right)^{1/2} \text{moles} \qquad [1]$$

$P_R^{180°}$ and $P_S^{180°}$ are the transmitter power into 50 Ω for a nonselective, 1-ms 180° inversion pulse on the phantom and subject respectively and reflect their relative "receive" sensitivities [37].

Note that although the WBNAA sequence obtains a full, whole-head ^{1}H spectrum, as shown in Fig. 1, it relies for localization on the prior knowledge that NAA is found only in neuronal cells, i.e., is intrinsically localized to the brain. Therefore, it cannot correctly quantify the brain's contribution to the other

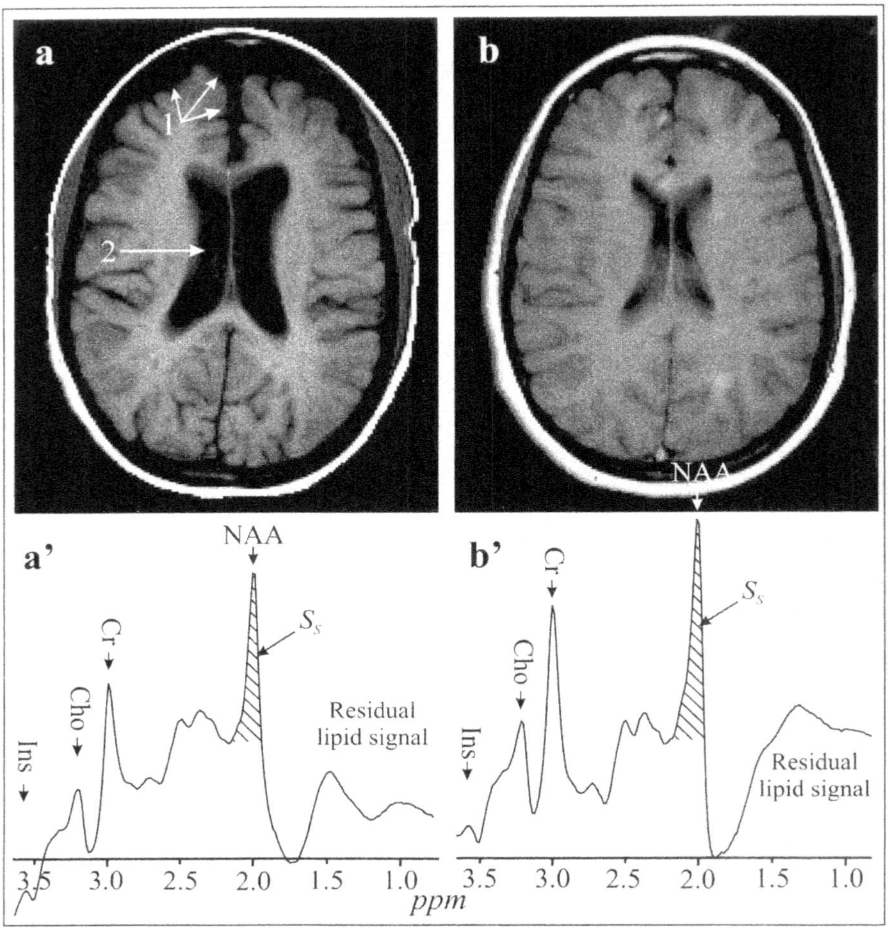

Fig. 1a, b. Corresponding axial T1-weighted MRI of a 28- and a 30-year-old woman with RRMS with respectively 6.5 and 0.25 years' disease duration, and both with an EDSS score of 1.5. Note the increased atrophy, reflected by enlarged subarachnoid spaces and cortical sulci (*1*) and lateral ventricles (*2*). **a'**, **b'** The whole-head ^{1}H spectra, on the same chemical shift and intensity scales, corrected for coil loading and V_B. The *hatched* regions indicate the S_S used to evaluate Q_{NAA} of Eq. 1. Note (1) the overall similarity of the spectral features, indicating cross-sectional reproducibility; (2) near-complete lipid suppression; and (3) lower NAA area in the patient with the longer disease duration, **a'** versus **b'**. Note also that although the sequence yields a complete whole-head ^{1}H spectrum, it relies on the prior knowledge that NAA is found only in neuronal cells. Therefore, it cannot quantify the brain's contribution to the other metabolites (Cho, Cr, mI, etc.) which are also present in other tissue types

metabolites (e.g., choline, creatine, Ins) peaks in the TE=0 ms spectrum, since these are also present in other tissue types in the head, e.g., muscle, subcutaneous lipids, and bone marrow. Consequently, the ensuing discussion will focus exclusively on NAA.

To account for normal intersubject head size variations, each Q_{NAA} was divided by the brain volume, V_B, of that individual to yield the subject's specific WBNAA concentration,

$$\text{WBNAA} = \frac{Q_{NAA}}{V_B}, \qquad [2]$$

which, since it is a normalized per-unit-volume metric, is independent of the brain volume and therefore suitable for cross-sectional, interindividual comparisons.

Statistical Analysis

A two-tailed Student t-test for nonpaired data was used to compare the patients' WBNAA levels and absolute and percentage GM and WM volumes with the controls'.

Results

The median T2LV in the patients was 5.5 cm^3 (range: 0.14-29.0). GM and WM comprised 50.4±3.8% and 30.4±5.0% (mean±standard deviation), respectively, of the total cranial volume, in the patients and 53.8±3.7% and 35.4±4.7% in the controls. The percentages of GM and WM were significantly lower in patients than in controls (p=0.047 and 0.029, respectively). GM and WM absolute volumes were significantly lower in patients than in the controls (p=0.046 and 0.006, respectively). Expressed as fractions of just the parenchyma, the GM and WM fractions were 60% and 40% for the controls versus 62% and 38% for the patients.

A significant difference was found between the average WBNAA level of the patients, $\overline{\text{WBNAA}^p}$ = 10.03 mM (range: 4.78-14.04 mM) and that of the controls, $\overline{\text{WBNAA}^c}$ = 12.90 mM (11.5-14.5 mM) (p<0.0001). To express the differences within and between the controls' and patients' populations in percentage rather than millimoles, we constructed the unitless metric Δ_{WBNAA} for the percentage of a subject's WBNAA level difference from the controls' average:

$$\Delta_{WBNA} = \frac{\text{WBNAA} - \overline{\text{WBNAA}^c}}{\overline{\text{WBNAA}^c}} \cdot 100\%. \qquad [3]$$

These values for each of the 41 controls in the study, Δ^c_{WBNAA}, are plotted in Fig. 2, as are the 71 patients' Δ^p_{WBNAA}. The *inter*subject variability of WBNAA, which has previously shown a standard deviation, σ, of 0.6 mM, (~5%) in controls [25], has exhibited a σ of 0.7 mM (~6%) in this 41-subject cohort. Compared with the controls' average $\overline{\Delta^c_{WBNAA}}$ (=0%), the patient's mean, $\overline{\Delta^p_{WBNAA}}$, was 22% lower (range +8% to –63%).

Discussion

Considering the standard deviation (σ=6%) variation of the WBNAA level in the controls, the patients in the shaded, $\overline{\Delta^p_{WBNAA}}$ ± 2σ (±12%), region of Fig. 2 are statistically indistinguishable from the healthy subjects in Fig. 2, whereas those outside are more than 95% likely to be different. Not surprisingly, of 71 MS patients, 48 (67%) are *below* that "normal" region. Even of the 23 patients inside that region, two-thirds are *below* average Δ^c_{WBNAA}, and none is above $+2\sigma$ (+12%). This is in contrast to the controls in Fig. 1, half of whom are above the average of 0% and half below.

T2WI lesion loads are reported to rarely exceed 3% of the brain volume in RRMS [26]. Since in our cohort they averaged less than 0.5% (maximum 2.9%), even complete axonal (NAA) loss in all the lesions would not statistically distinguish a patient's WBNAA level from the controls. Consequently, deficits upwards of 3%, whether reversible in part, as sometimes suggested, [38, 39] or not, must implicate NAWM [22]. Since the sensitivity of the WBNAA method is of the order of ±6%, any loss greater than 6% is therefore significant and must involve not only lesions (which comprise less than 3% of the brain volume) but NAWM as well. Given that in our patient cohort the WM comprises approximately 37% of the parenchymal volume [27] and its NAA concentration is approximately two-thirds of the GM's [28], extending the above argument suggests that Δ^p_{WBNAA} below $2/3 \times 37\%_W = {}_W{-25\%}$ cannot be accounted for even by complete NAA depletion in the WM and lesions. However, since patients whose Δ^p_{WBNAA} is above −12% (-2σ) are formally statistically indistinguishable from the controls, "true deficits" were attributed only from the −12% lower edge of the latter distribution rather than its center, as shown in Fig. 2.

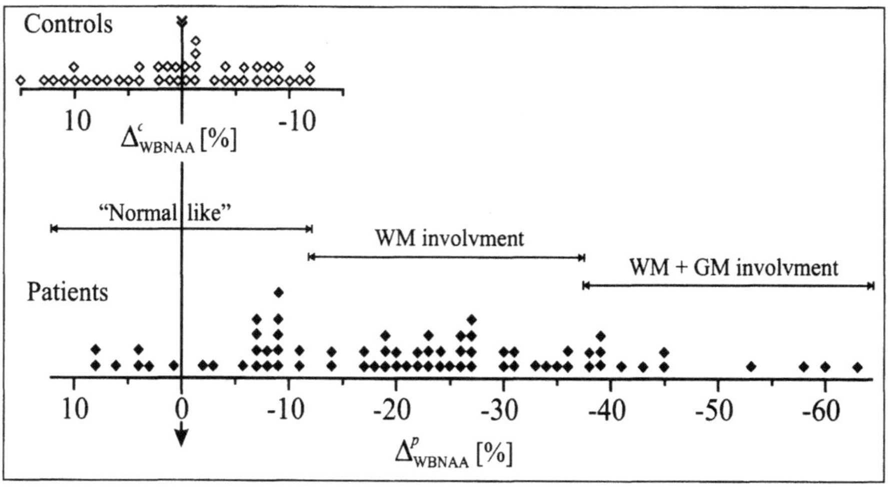

Fig. 2. *Top:* Dot plot of the 41 healthy controls' Δ^c_{WBNAA} [%] from Eq. 3, Δ^c_{WBNAA} ◇, whose average $\overline{\Delta^c_{WBNAA}}$, was 0% (*vertical arrow*). *Bottom:* Same for the 71 MS patients' Δ^p_{WBNAA} [%], ◆, whose average $\overline{\Delta^p_{WBNAA}}$, was −22%. Those inside the $\overline{\Delta^c_{WBNAA}} \pm 2\sigma$ (±12%) zone are statistically indistinguishable from the controls and labeled "normal-like". The $-12\% \geq \Delta^p_{WBNAA} \geq 37\%$ region highlights patients whose NAA deficit can be accounted for by lesions and NAWM involvement. Higher deficits ($\Delta^p_{WBNAA} \leq -37\%$) cannot, and therefore must implicate GM as well

Even this conservative cutoff left 48 of the 71 patients' WBNAA below the "normal-like" range. Of these, the 35 in the "WM involvement" zone of Fig. 2 have sustained losses that can be explained by WM deficits, whereas the 13 in the "WM+GM involvement" region suffered Δ^{P}_{WBNAA} more than 25% below the lowest "normal" of −12%, i.e., true-deficits greater than −37%, exceeding the entire NAA content of their WM. Nevertheless, these 13 had the same average disease duration of 4.9 (range 2-10) years as the rest. Furthermore, this cohort exhibited only slight clinical disability, reflected by relatively low average EDSS scores of 2.0, an additional indication of relative overall WM integrity. Therefore, although WBNAA yields just the global concentration, not localized levels and not even WM versus GM fractions, upwards of 25% deficits *must* be distributed over the *whole* brain, including substantial portions of GM.

It is noteworthy that although axonal damage has been reported in classical neuropathology for over a century, only recently have postmortem studies shown that neurons are also targets of the MS process [4, 15, 40-42] and that their dysfunction may contribute to clinical disability [14, 41]. Indeed, Peterson et al. reported that cerebral cortex MS lesions are characterized by demyelination, axonal and dendritic transection, and apoptotic loss of neurons [15]. In addition, subcortical lesions which result in axonal transection might be accompanied by retrograde neuronal degeneration. Unfortunately, such lesions are frequently missed by both conventional T2WI, due to their small size, poor contrast with surrounding GM, and partial volume effects with adjacent WM [14]; and by pathology, which inspects only a few small tissue samples, usually obtained post mortem. Consequently, several important parameters pertaining to GM involvement, e.g., time of onset, location, and the extent of neuronal damage, are uncertain.

Since all the patients in this study are in their initial, only mildly disabled, RR stage, the finding that nearly 20% of them already display sufficient NAA loss to implicate their GM may indicate that neuronal damage may be an early consequence of the MS process. As for the conjugate issues of its location(s) and extent: 10% GM involvement and higher indicates that lesion density similar to the WM's (<3%) is insufficient to explain such profound NAA decline. This finding is consistent with a recent report of approximately 20% average WBNAA decrease in patients at the earliest clinical stage of MS, who typically show negligible (<1%) lesion volumes [43]. Therefore, in analogy with NAWM axonal pathology, substantial diffuse neuronal dysfunction in the GM must also be assumed. This concept is also corroborated by recent MTI and DTI studies showing differences between the magnetization transfer ratio and mean diffusivity histograms from the GM of MS patients compared with matched controls [16, 19], suggesting subtle diffuse tissue damage. However, since MTI and DTI reflect structural abnormalities, increased extracellular water and loss of barriers to its motion, neither are as specific to neuronal (NAA) loss or cover as extensive a brain fraction as WBNAA.

Focal Metabolic Evidence of Deep GM Involvement

Introduction

As outlined under "Global Evidence of Grey Matter Involvement" above, after 130 years of being considered a WM disease, the GM involvement at cortical and subcortical level in MS is now gaining increased recognition [15, 42]. Since the thalami and basal ganglia are critical links of a cortical-subcortical circuit controlling several neurological domains, their injury or dysfunction may lead to sensorimotor, cerebellar, and cognitive deficits as well as fatigue [44]. Yet, despite mounting postmortem evidence [13], most of the T2WI, MTI, and DTI studies have so far failed to detect significant abnormalities of the basal ganglia in MS patients in vivo [45].

^{1}H-MRS facilitates noninvasive assessment of neurons, axons, and membrane integrity through the quantification of NAA, total choline (Cho) and creatine (Cr) levels. Decreased NAA coupled with Cho and Cr variations has been reported in MS lesions, NAWM, and cortical GM [46]. Such diffuse pathology naturally lends itself to multivoxel acquisition of large brain volumes in order to quantify the distribution of metabolites in several bilateral structures in one study [46]. While thalamic neurodegeneration in MS investigated with histopathology and in vivo ^{1}H-MRS has been described recently, the single-voxel method used excluded the basal ganglia [47]. This elegant study motivated us to use 3D ^{1}H-MRS to compare the metabolite levels of several deep GM nuclei of RRMS patients with those of controls and investigate their relationship with the patients' neurological deficits.

Methods

Subjects

Eleven RRMS patients (8 women), mean age 39 years (range: 26-48 years), and 9 healthy controls (7 women), mean age 38 years (range: 21-48 years), were studied. The median disease duration was 6.9 years (3.9-10.9 years), median EDSS score was 2.5 (0.0-6.0), and median pyramidal and sensory functional system (FS) scores were 1.0 (0.0-3.0) and 0.0 (0.0-2.0) respectively. All subjects were briefed on the procedures they were about to undertake and gave their written Institutional Review Board-approved informed consent.

MRI and Quantitative 3D ^{1}H-MRS

MRI and 3D ^{1}H-MRS were performed in a 1.5-T imager (Magnetom 63SP, Siemens AG, Erlangen, Germany). Contiguous axial, sagittal, and coronal T_1-weighted (T1WI) spin-echo (TE/TR=15/450 ms) and axial T2WI dual spin-echo ($TE_1/TE_2/TR$=16/90/2500 ms) 7.5-mm-thick slices were obtained at 240×240 mm^2 field of view and 256×256 matrix. A 3D ^{1}H-MRS sequence TE/TR=135/1600 ms followed. It excited an image-guided $8_{LR}\times10_{AP}\times6_{IS}$ cm^3 left-right (LR) × anterior-posterior (AP) × inferior-superior (IS) volume of interest

(VOI) centered on the corpus callosum, as shown in Fig. 3. That VOI was partitioned into $8_{LR}\times10_{AP}\times8_{IS}$=640 voxels, 0.75 cm^3 each [46]. The MRS part of the protocol took 54 min and the entire exam was completed in less than 80 min.

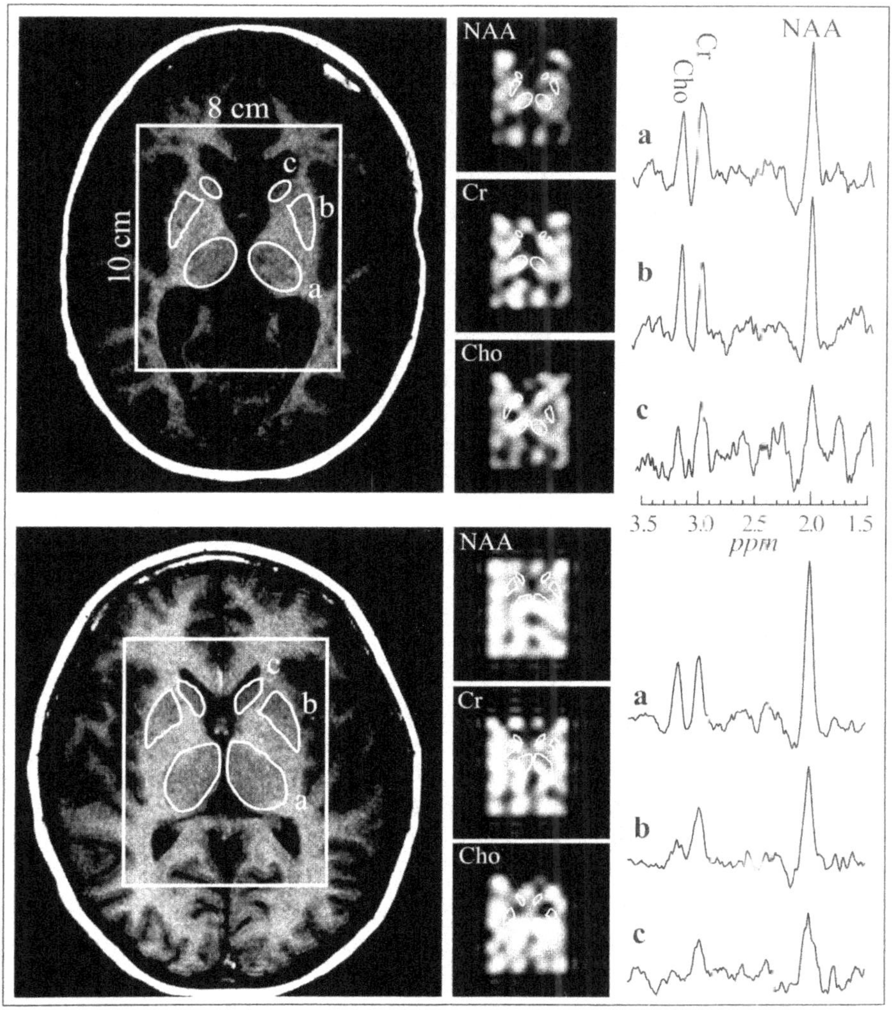

Fig. 3. *Top:* T1WI of an axial slice in the brain of a 28-year-old woman with RRMS from a level containing **a** the thalamus, **b** putamen head of the caudate, and **c** (*left*), with the $8_{LR}\times10_{AP}$ cm^2 VOI (*solid box*) and the manually outlined nuclei superimposed. *Center:* NAA, Cr, and Cho metabolic maps from the VOI with the corresponding nuclei outlines from the image transcribed. *Right:* Average ^{1}H spectra from each of the labeled nuclei. *Bottom:* Same as top for a matched control. Metabolic maps and spectra are drawn on the same chemical shift (horizontal) and intensity scales. Note the general trends to higher NAA and lower Cho peaks in the spectra from the deep nuclei of the control

The MRS data was zero-filled from 1024 to 2048 points in the time and 16×16 to 128×128 in the spatial domains, reconstructed, frequency-aligned, and phase-corrected in each voxel [46]. Relative NAA, Cr, and Cho levels were estimated from their peak areas using parametric spectral modeling and least-squares optimization [48]. This software accommodates spectral line shifts and broadening which could result from increased iron contents due to both normal aging as well as pathological processes and which could lead to susceptibility and T2 broadening in the deep GM nuclei studied. These relative amounts of metabolites were scaled into absolute levels, $[Q]$, in each voxel by phantom replacement with a 3-l sphere of 10.9 mM NAA in water [49] as described for Eq. [1] above. These levels were corrected for the difference between the in vitro NAA: T_1^{vitro}/T_2^{vitro}=1.4/0.75 s and those reported for in vivo NAA: 1.4/0.43 s, Cr: 1.6/0.21 s, and Cho: 1.2/0.36 s in each voxel using [49]:

$$[Q] \approx Q(\text{vitro}) \cdot \left(1 - \frac{TE \cdot (T_{2j}^{vivo} - T_{2j}^{vitro})}{T_{2j}^{vivo} - T_{2j}^{vitro}}\right) \cdot \frac{T_1^{vitro}}{T_1^{vivo}} \text{mM}. \qquad [4]$$

This calculation ignores possible regional and tissue T_1/T_2 variations [50, 51]. However, we do not believe that this will significantly affect the results since: (1) We compared voxels in similar anatomical positions; and (2) for 90° nutation at TR=1.2×T_1 the signal is relatively insensitive to T_1 differences, with a change of ±20% in T_1 giving only a ±5% change in signal [52].

To avoid partial CSF volume effects, only voxels completely within a nucleus, with no apparent ventricular or sulcal involvement, were considered. Therefore, no correction was made for possible increased extracellular water such as that described by Helms [53].

Statistical Analyses

Mixed model analysis of variance was conducted to test the effect of disease state (patient versus controls), laterality (left versus right), and age on each metabolite level while accommodating the correlations introduced by the acquisition of multiple metabolite assessments per subject. Spearman rank correlation coefficients were used to estimate the strength of the association of disease duration, age, EDSS, and pyramidal and sensory FS scores with the metabolite levels of the patients. Due to the correlation of metabolite assessments from the same subject, the significance of the associations was assessed using mixed model analysis of variance.

Results

No T2WI or T1WI lesions were detected in the deep GM nuclei of the patients. Age was not associated with [NAA], [Cr], or [Cho]. Since the level differences between nuclei on the left and right sides of patients or controls was insignificant, only their averages are given in Table 1. The mean [NAA] in these nuclei was lower and [Cho] higher in patients than in controls (p<0.02 for both),

Table 1. Mean±standard deviation of NAA, Cho, and Cr millimolar concentrations (mM) in the deep GM of RRMS patients and controls

	RRMS	Controls	*p*
[NAA]	8.85±2.18	9.50±1.97	<0.02
[Cr]	6.43±1.53	6.51±1.62	n.s.
[Cho]	2.16±0.55	1.86±0.47	<0.02

whereas no significant difference was found for the [Cr]. While the [NAA] was associated with sensory FS score (p=0.01), the metabolite levels correlated with neither the patients' disease duration nor their EDSS scores.

For each subject, an axial T1WI showing the thalamus, head of caudate, and putamen and the three corresponding metabolic maps (NAA, Cr and Cho) were chosen, as shown in Fig. 1. The thalami and basal ganglia were manually outlined on the image using our custom software, which also transcribed them onto the corresponding regions of the three metabolic maps. The program then computed the average spectrum, metabolite levels, and their standard deviation from each outlined region (cf. Fig. 1).

Discussion

Unlike cortical GM, the deep nuclei are technically easier to access with ^{1}H-MRS. To probe their metabolism we used high-spatial-resolution (1 cm interpolated to 0.125 cm in-plane) 3D ^{1}H-MRS to minimize contamination from CSF or the surrounding WM. Still, due to their smaller size and less well-defined borders, the head of the caudate and the putamen were less straightforward to delineate than the much larger thalamus (cf. Fig. 1).

Most of the MRI studies which investigated the basal ganglia with MTI and DTI did not find abnormalities. Nevertheless, it is well known that different subpopulations of striatal neurons are differentially compromised in acute and chronic neurological disease [54] and that basal ganglia of MS patients suffer from glucose hypometabolism [55]. Therefore, our observation of significant [NAA] reduction in the deep GM of these RRMS patients compared to their controls is consistent with a recent study suggesting that neuronal loss occurs in thalamic GM from the earliest stages of MS [47].

The approximately 7% [NAA] decrease in the patients' nuclei is similar to that reported in a large (0.5 l) volume of NAWM in the same cohort, whereas the 14% [Cho] elevation is less than half and the [Cr] unchanged compared with the controls' [49]. While the NAA decrease is probably due to Wallerian degeneration of GM neurons secondary to the damage of fibers traversing MS white matter lesions, and/or to local microscopic foci of inflammation [47], a smaller Cho increase is not entirely unexpected considering that the nuclei studied contain approximately 3-5% myelin versus 24% in WM. We speculate that a decline in NAA without a concomitant increase in Cr might reflect either neuronal dysfunction or an initial loss without a (yet) significant replacement with glial cells.

Interestingly, not only is the deep GM not spared by MS, but it has a higher estimated number of lesions per gram wet weight than any other brain structure [13]. Unfortunately, the lesions are frequently missed on T2WI due to their small size and poor contrast with the surrounding GM. These lesions along with the glucose hypometabolism documented in the basal ganglia of MS patients [55] are probably responsible for the increase in Cho level observed in this patient cohort.

Finally, we did not find any correlation between metabolite levels in these nuclei and either disease duration or EDSS scores. The latter is not surprising considering the known limitations of that scale and the narrow range of disability in our patients. Nonetheless, the NAA decline did correlate with the sensory impairment, as expected from the central role of the thalamus as a relay for sensory pathways that are very often involved in MS. Future studies should, therefore, include extensive cognitive tests and fatigue rating scale to associate the clinical aspects of the disease with its metabolic aspects.

Conclusions

Our observations, both indirect under "Global Evidence of Grey Matter Involvement" and direct under "Focal Metabolic Evidence of Deep GM Involvement", are consistent with previous ^{1}H-MRS studies showing significant NAA reduction in GM of patients with early RRMS [17, 18, 42, 47, 56] and with a functional PET study showing that GM hypometabolism worsens over time [57]. The contribution of accumulating GM damage to WBNAA decline is supported by its lower volume in our patients relative to their controls, and is consistent with other recent findings [58, 59], and may be responsible for, or contribute to, frequent clinical manifestation of cognitive impairment [60]. Finally, the direct and indirect evidence presented suggests that RRMS is not exclusively a WM disease. Rather, it may need to be reclassified as a "diffuse whole-brain disorder." This increases the motivation to validate surrogate markers for early axonal/neuronal damage in order to identify high risk of neurodegeneration, and underscores the need to develop treatments to not only reduce inflammation, but also to restore, preserve, and protect the normal neuronal environment.

Acknowledgements. The authors are grateful to the study's patient coordinator Ms. Lois J. Mannon, RT, and to our collaborators, Drs. Belinda S. Y. Li, Yulin Ge, Juan He, Andrew A. Maudsley, Brian J. Soher, and James S. Babb. This work was supported by the Fondazione Italiana Sclerosi Multipla (MI) and NIH grants EB01015, NS37739, and NS29029.

References

1. Charcot J (1868) Histologie de le sclérose en plaques. Gaz Hop (Paris) 141:554-555, 557-558
2. Arnold DL, Matthews PM, Francis G, Antel J (1990) Proton magnetic resonance spectroscopy of human brain in vivo in the evaluation of multiple sclerosis: assessment of the load of disease. Magn Reson Med 14:154-159
3. Davie CA, Hawkins CP, Barker GJ et al (1994) Serial proton magnetic resonance spectroscopy in acute multiple sclerosis lesions. Brain 117:49-58
4. Trapp BD, Peterson J, Ransohoff RM et al (1998) Axonal transection in the lesions of multiple sclerosis. N Engl J Med 338:278-285
5. van Walderveen MA, Barkhof F, Pouwels PJ et al (1999) Neuronal damage in T1-hypointense multiple sclerosis lesions demonstrated in vivo using proton magnetic resonance spectroscopy. Ann Neurol 46:79-87
6. Allen IV, McKeown SR (1979) A histological, histochemical and biochemical study of the macroscopically normal white matter in multiple sclerosis. J Neurol Sci 41:81-91
7. Evangelou N, Esiri MM, Smith S et al (2000) Quantitative pathological evidence for axonal loss in normal appearing white matter in multiple sclerosis. Ann Neurol 47:391-395
8. Miki Y, Grossman RI, Udupa JK et al (1999) Differences between relapsing-remitting and chronic progressive multiple sclerosis as determined with quantitative MR imaging. Radiology 210:769-774
9. Loevner LA, Grossman RI, Cohen JA et al (1995) Microscopic disease in normal-appearing white matter on conventional MR images in patients with multiple sclerosis: assessment with magnetization-transfer measurements. Radiology 196:511-515
10. Filippi M, Cercignani M, Inglese M et al (2001) Diffusion tensor magnetic resonance imaging in multiple sclerosis. Neurology 56:304-311
11. Fu L, Matthews PM, De Stefano N et al (1998) Imaging axonal damage of normal-appearing white matter in multiple sclerosis. Brain 121:103-113
12. Brownell B, Hughes J (1962) The distribution of plaques in the cerebrum in multiple sclerosis. J Neurol Neurosurg Psychiatry 25:315-320
13. Lumsden C (1970) The neuropathology of multiple sclerosis. In: Vinken Pj BG (ed) Handbook of clinical neurology. North-Holland, Amsterdam, p 217-309
14. Kidd D, Barkhof F, McConnell R et al (1999) Cortical lesions in multiple sclerosis. Brain 122:17-26
15. Peterson JW, Bo L, Mork S et al (2001) Transected neurites, apoptotic neurons, and reduced inflammation in cortical multiple sclerosis lesions. Ann Neurol 50:389-400
16. Ge Y, Grossman RI, Udupa JK et al (2001) Magnetization transfer ratio histogram analysis of grey matter in relapsing-remitting multiple sclerosis. AJNR Am J Neuroradiol 22:470-475
17. Kapeller P, McLean MA, Griffin CM et al (2001) Preliminary evidence for neuronal damage in cortical grey matter and normal appearing white matter in short duration relapsing-remitting multiple sclerosis: a quantitative MR spectroscopic imaging study. J Neurol 248:131-138
18. Sharma R, Narayana PA, Wolinsky JS (2001) Grey matter abnormalities in multiple sclerosis: proton magnetic resonance spectroscopic imaging. Mult Scler 7:221-226
19. Bozzali M, Cercignani M, Sormani MP et al (2002) Quantification of brain grey matter damage in different MS phenotypes by use of diffusion tensor MR imaging. AJNR Am J Neuroradiol 23:985-988
20. Simmons ML, Frondoza CG, Coyle JT (1991) Immunocytochemical localization of *N*-acetyl-aspartate with monoclonal antibodies. Neuroscience 45:37-45
21. Matthews PM, Pioro E, Narayanan S et al (1996) Assessment of lesion pathology in

multiple sclerosis using quantitative MRI morphometry and magnetic resonance spectroscopy. Brain 119:715-722
22. Gonen O, Catalaa I, Babb JS et al (2000) Total brain *N*-acetylaspartate: a new measure of disease load in MS. Neurology 54:15-19
23. De Stefano N, Narayanan S, Mortilla M et al (2000) Imaging axonal damage in multiple sclerosis by means of MR spectroscopy. Neurol Sci 21:S883-887
24. Li BS, Babb JS, Soher BJ et al (2002) Reproducibility of 3D proton spectroscopy in the human brain. Magn Reson Med 47:439-446
25. Gonen O, Viswanathan AK, Catalaa I et al (1998) Total brain *N*-acetylaspartate concentration in normal, age-grouped females: Quantitation with non-echo proton NMR spectroscopy. Magn Reson Med 40:684-689
26. Miki Y, Grossman RI, Udupa JK et al (1999) Relapsing-remitting multiple sclerosis: longitudinal analysis of MR images-lack of correlation between changes in T2 lesion volume and clinical findings. Radiology 213:395-399
27. Courchesne E, Chisum HJ, Townsend J et al (2000) Normal brain development and aging: quantitative analysis at in vivo MR imaging in healthy volunteers. Radiology 216:672-682
28. Wang Y, Li SJ (1998) Differentiation of metabolic concentrations between grey matter and white matter of human brain by in vivo 1H magnetic resonance spectroscopy. Magn Reson Med 39:28-33
29. Lublin FD, Reingold SC (1996) Defining the clinical course of multiple sclerosis: results of an international survey. National Multiple Sclerosis Society (USA) Advisory Committee on Clinical Trials of New Agents in Multiple Sclerosis. Neurology 46:907-911
30. Kurtzke JF (1983) Rating neurologic impairment in multiple sclerosis: an expanded disability status scale (EDSS). Neurology 33:1444-1452
31. Udupa JK, Odhner D, Samarasekera S (1994) 3DVIEWNIX: an open, transportable, multdimensional, multimodality, multiparametric imging software system. Proc SPIE 2164:58-73
32. Udupa JK, Samarasekera S (1996) Fuzzy connectedness and object definition: theory, algorithms, and applications in image segmentation. Graph Models Image Process 58:246-261
33. Ge Y, Grossman RI, Udupa JK et al (2000) Brain atrophy in relapsing-remitting multiple sclerosis and secondary progressive multiple sclerosis: longitudinal quantitative analysis. Radiology 214:665-670
34. Udupa JK, Wei L, Miki Y, Grossman RI (1997) A system for the comprehensive analysis of multiple sclerosis lesion load based on MR imagery [abstract]. In: Proceedings of the Society of Photo-Optical Instrumentation Engineers program. Newport Beach, Calif, pp 610-618
35. Samarasekera S, Udupa JK, Miki Y et al (1997) A new computer-assisted method for the quantification of enhancing lesions in multiple sclerosis. J Comput Assist Tomogr 21:145-151
36. Soher BJ, van Zijl PC, Duyn JH, Barker PB (1996) Quantitative proton MR spectroscopic imaging of the human brain. Magn Reson Med 35:356-363
37. Hoult DI, Richards RE (1976) The signal-to-noise ratio of the nuclear magnetic resonance experiment. J Magn Reson 24:71-85
38. Arnold DL, De Stefano N, Narayanan S, Matthews PM (2000) Proton MR spectroscopy in multiple sclerosis. Neuroimaging Clin North Am 10:789-798, ix-x
39. Narayana PA, Doyle TJ, Lai D, Wolinsky JS (1998) Serial proton magnetic resonance spectroscopic imaging, contrast-enhanced magnetic resonance imaging, and quantitative lesion volumetry in multiple sclerosis. Ann Neurol 43:56-71
40. Bjartmar C, Kidd G, Mork S et al (2000) Neurological disability correlates with spinal cord axonal loss and reduced *N*-acetyl aspartate in chronic multiple sclerosis patients. Ann Neurol 48:893-901

41. Bjartmar C, Kinkel RP, Kidd G et al (2001) Axonal loss in normal-appearing white matter in a patient with acute MS. Neurology 57:1248-1252
42. Cifelli A, Arridge M, Jezzard P et al (2002) Thalamic neurodegeneration in multiple sclerosis. Ann Neurol 52:650-653
43. Filippi M, Bozzali M, Rovaris M et al (2003) Evidence for widespread axonal damage at the earliest clinical stage of multiple sclerosis. Brain 126:433-437
44. Martin WRW, Snow B, Ashforth R (1999) Abnormalities of movement and posture due to disease of the extrapyramidal motor system. In: Greenberg JO (eds) Neuroimaging-a companion to Adams and Victor's principles of neurology. McGraw-Hill, New York
45. Filippi M, Bozzali M, Comi G (2001) Magnetization transfer and diffusion tensor MR imaging of basal ganglia from patients with multiple sclerosis. J Neurol Sci 183:69-72
46. Gonen O, Grossman RI (2001) New magnetic resonance spectroscopy strategies. In: Comi G (ed) Magnetic resonance spectroscopy in multiple sclerosis. Springer, Milan, pp 97-112
47. Wylezinska M, Cifelli A, Jezzard P et al (2003) Thalamic neurodegeneration in relapsing-remitting multiple sclerosis. Neurology 60:1949-1954
48. Soher BJ, Young K, Govindaraju V, Maudsley AA (1998) Automated spectral analysis III: Application to in vivo proton MR spectroscopy and spectroscopic imaging. Magn Reson Med 40:822-831
49. Inglese M, Li BS, Rusinek H et al (2003) Diffusely elevated cerebral choline and creatine in relapsing-remitting multiple sclerosis. Magn Reson Med 50:190-195
50. Kreis R, Ernst T, Ross BD (1993) Absolute concentrations of water and metabolites in the human brain. II. Metabolite concentrations. J Magn Reson 102:9-19
51. Christiansen P, Toft P, Larsson HB et al (1993) The concentration of *N*-acetyl aspartate, creatine + phosphocreatine, and choline in different parts of the brain in adulthood and senium. Magn Reson Imaging 11:799-806
52. Ernst RR, Bodenhausen G, Wokaun A (1987) Principles of nuclear magnetic resonance in one and two dimensions. Clarendon Press, Oxford, p 152
53. Helms G (2001) Volume correction for edema in single-volume proton MR spectroscopy of contrast-enhancing multiple sclerosis lesions. Magn Reson Med 46:256-263
54. Calabresi P, Centonze D, Bernardi G (2000) Cellular factors controlling neuronal vulnerability in the brain: a lesson from the striatum. Neurology 55:1249-1255
55. Roelcke U, Kappos L, Lechner-Scott J et al (1997) Reduced glucose metabolism in the frontal cortex and basal ganglia of multiple sclerosis patients with fatigue: a 18F-fluorodeoxyglucose positron emission tomography study. Neurology 48:1566-1571
56. Chard DT, Griffin CM, McLean MA et al (2002) Brain metabolite changes in cortical grey and normal-appearing white matter in clinically early relapsing-remitting multiple sclerosis. Brain 125:2342-2352
57. Blinkenberg M, Rune K, Jensen CV et al (2000) Cortical cerebral metabolism correlates with MRI lesion load and cognitive dysfunction in MS. Neurology 54:558-564
58. Chard DT, Griffin CM, Parker GJ et al (2002) Brain atrophy in clinically early relapsing-remitting multiple sclerosis. Brain 125:327-337
59. De Stefano N, Matthews PM, Filippi M et al (2003) Evidence of early cortical atrophy in MS: relevance to white matter changes and disability. Neurology 60:1157-1162
60. Rao SM, Leo GJ, Bernardin L, Unverzagt F (1991) Cognitive dysfunction in multiple sclerosis. I. Frequency, patterns, and prediction. Neurology 41:685-691

Chapter 13

Functional MRI in Multiple Sclerosis*

M. Filippi, M.A. Rocca

Introduction

During the last decade, important efforts have been devoted to improving our understanding of the pathophysiology of multiple sclerosis (MS), with the ultimate goal of identifying and monitoring treatment strategies with the potential to modify the evolution of the disease favorably. One of the major results of this increased research interest in MS is that the classical notion of MS as a demyelinating disease affecting the white matter of the central nervous system (CNS) has been challenged significantly. First, it became apparent that axonal pathology in macroscopic brain lesions and normal-appearing brain tissue (NABT) is an important aspect of the disease from its earliest phases [1-3]. Second, it was shown that grey matter is not spared by the disease [4-10]. Finally, brain plasticity is now considered an important factor which might contribute to the clinical recovery and the maintenance of a normal level of function in the presence of irreversible axonal/neuronal loss.

In this chapter, the main functional MRI (fMRI) studies performed in patients with MS are summarized to show how they are changing our views of the ability of the brain in MS to limit the clinical consequences of irreversible structural tissue damage.

What Does fMRI Measure?

The signal changes seen during fMRI studies depend on the blood oxygenation level-dependent (BOLD) mechanism, which, in turn, involves changes of the transverse magnetization relaxation time – either T_2* in a gradient echo sequence, or T_2 in a spin echo sequence [11, 12]. Local increases in neuronal activity result in a rise in blood flow and oxygen consumption. The increase in blood flow is greater than the increase in oxygen consumption, thus bringing about an increased ratio between oxygenated and deoxygenated hemoglobin, which enhances the MRI signal [11, 12]. As these signal changes are very modest (usually ranging from 0.5% to 1.5%), it is usually

---

* This chapter represents an update of the chapter by the same authors entitled "Functional MRI", in *New Frontiers of MR-Based Techniques in Multiple Sclerosis*, edited by M. Filippi and G. Comi (Springer, Milan, 2003), pp 83–97

necessary to obtain a large number of brain images acquired during alternated periods of activation (motor, sensory, and cognitive) and rest. As a consequence, concern has been raised regarding intersubject and intersession variability in the fMRI signal. However, by analyzing these data with appropriate statistical methods, it is possible to obtain information about the location and the extent of specific areas involved in the performance of a given task in healthy subjects and in patients with different neurological conditions [13, 14].

Early fMRI Studies in MS

The main problem in the interpretation of fMRI studies is that the observed changes might be biased by differences in task performance between patients and controls. Clearly, this is a major issue in MS which typically causes impairment of various functional systems. Although this might have limited the value of the earliest fMRI studies of patients with MS [15-21], they provide several important pieces of information, which can be summarized as follows:

1. Cortical reorganization is likely to be an early phenomenon in the course of MS. A study of the visual system [17] in patients who had recovered from a single episode of acute optic neuritis demonstrated that such patients (compared to healthy volunteers) had extensive activation of the visual network (including the claustrum, lateral temporal and posterior parietal cortices, and thalamus, in addition to the primary visual cortex). Furthermore, the volume of the extraoccipital activation in patients with optic neuritis was found to correlate strongly with the latency of the visual evoked potentials (VEP), suggesting that the functional reorganization of the cortex might represent an adaptive response to a persistently abnormal visual input.
2. Functional cortical changes might have a dynamic behavior related to the clinical manifestations and the underlying pathological substrates [15, 18]. Using a simple motor task, two studies found prominent changes in the recruitment of the contralateral and ipsilateral primary sensorimotor cortex (SMC) and supplementary motor area (SMA) during recovery from an acute relapse in patients with relapsing-remitting (RR) MS. In one of these studies, a strong correlation was found between the extent of functional cortical changes and *N*-acetylaspartate (NAA) levels [18], indicating that dynamic reorganization of the motor cortex can occur in response to an axonal injury associated with MS activity.
3. Adaptive functional changes in the cerebral cortex have been described in patients with RRMS and secondary progressive (SP) MS for the visual [19, 20] and motor [16, 21] systems and have been variously related to clinical disability and to disease burden, measured using conventional MRI [16] and proton MR spectroscopy (^{1}H-MRS) [21].

Recent fMRI Studies in MS

fMRI in Patients with Clinically Isolated Syndromes Suggestive of MS

The first manifestation of MS is, in many cases, an acute, remitting, clinically isolated syndrome (CIS) involving the optic nerves, brainstem, or spinal cord [22]. Recent quantitative MRI studies have shown that irreversible tissue loss can occur in these patients [23-25], as well as in those with early RRMS [26, 27], despite the absence or paucity of clinical manifestations outside of the acute phases. To investigate better how early cortical reorganization occurs in the course of MS and its role in limiting the clinical outcome of the disease, fMRI has been used to study the visual and the motor systems of patients with CIS suggestive of MS [28-33].

Two studies of the visual system in patients with a single episode of optic neuritis [28, 29] extended the findings of Werring et al. [17]. In particular, Toosy et al. [28] replicated a previous study [17], using a longer photic stimulation epoch to better elucidate the nature of the abnormal extraoccipital response observed. The results of this study confirmed the original finding, suggesting that cortical functional changes might have a role in compensating for a persistently disordered visual input. Russ et al. [29] used fMRI and VEP to monitor functional recovery after an acute episode of unilateral optic neuritis and found a strong relationship between fMRI and VEP latencies, suggesting that fMRI might contribute to the assessment of the temporal evolution of the visual deficits during MS recovery or therapy.

fMRI has also been used to study, within 3 months from the first clinical relapse, the movement-associated cortical activations in patients at presentation with CIS highly suggestive of MS [30, 31], and to investigate the relationship between the extent of cortical activations and the extent of overall brain axonal pathology, measured using an unlocalized ^{1}H-MRS technique [30]. Compared to healthy controls, CIS patients had an altered brain pattern of movement-associated cortical activations, characterized by increased recruitment of the contralateral primary SMC during the performance of simple tasks [30, 31] and by the recruitment of additional "classical" and "higher-order" sensorimotor areas during the performance of more complex tasks [31]. CIS patients also had significantly reduced whole-brain NAA (WBNAA) concentrations. Interestingly, a strong inverse correlation was found between the extent of the contralateral primary SMC recruitment and the WBNAA concentration, suggesting that functional cortical reorganization might contribute to the maintenance of normal functional capacities from the earliest clinical stage of MS.

Pantano et al. [32] studied a group of patients with early MS diagnosed according to the McDonald criteria [34] and with a previous episode of hemiparesis. Using a simple motor task, they found that patients had increased activation of several cortical areas, mainly located in the ipsilateral hemisphere. Since the patients included in this study had had a previous hemiparesis, this did not allow interference of task performance on the results to be completely ruled out [32], and consequently these authors extended their investigations to a group of patients who had had a previous episode of optic neuritis [33]. They found that, during right-hand movement, cortical activation in optic neuritis patients was mainly in the contralateral hemisphere, whereas in patients with a previous hemiparesis, increased motor system recruitment was bilateral, with marked activation of areas located in the ipsilateral hemisphere. The extent of the ipsilateral activations in these patients correlated with the lesion damage in the corticospinal tracts [33].

fMRI in Patients with RRMS and no Clinical Disability

Despite the presence of irreversible axonal damage [1-3, 23-25], quite a large number of patients with RRMS experience relapses and accumulation of MRI lesion burden without being left with any major residual neurological deficits. To understand better whether adaptive cortical reorganization has a role in limiting the impact of irreversible tissue loss in these patients, a study has investigated the brain pattern of cortical activations during the performance of a simple motor task in nondisabled RRMS patients [35]. In this study, the magnitude of the correlation between fMRI changes and the extent of T_2-visible lesions, as well as the severity of MS pathology in lesions and NABT, measured using magnetization transfer MRI (MTI) and diffusion tensor MRI (DTI), were also investigated. Compared to healthy controls, MS patients showed increased activation of several regions mainly located in the contralateral cerebral hemisphere, including the primary SMC, the secondary somatosensory cortex (SII) and the intraparietal sulcus (IPS). In addition, they also showed increased bilateral activation of the SMA and the cingulate motor area (CMA). Strong correlations were found between the extent of fMRI activations and several MTI and DTI metrics of structural brain damage. This study demonstrated that cortical activation occurs over a rather distributed sensorimotor network in nondisabled RRMS patients, and provided additional evidence that increased recruitment of this cortical network contributes to limiting the functional impact of MS damage associated with macroscopic lesions and subtle NABT changes. Interestingly, in a group of patients with clinical characteristics similar to those recruited in the previous study, but who complained of fatigue, reduced activation of a complex movement-associated cortical/subcortical network including the cerebellum, the central operculum, the thalamus, and the middle frontal gyrus (MFG) was demonstrated in comparison to matched nonfatigued MS patients [36]. A strong correlation between the reduction of thalamic activity and the severity of fatigue was also found [36]. This suggests that reduced brain recruitment might be associated with the appearance of MS symptomatology.

fMRI in Patients with RRMS and SPMS and Mild to Moderate Clinical Disability

Since subtle damage of the NABT is an established feature of RRMS [7-9, 37], the impact of NABT damage, assessed using DTI, on movement-associated fMRI activations in patients with RRMS and nonspecific T_2-weighted abnormalities on conventional MRI of the brain has been investigated [38]. To assess the role of the nondominant hemisphere and interhemispheric connections on the dominant hand movement-associated pattern of activations, patients were studied during the performance of simple motor tasks with the dominant and the nondominant hand. Compared to healthy volunteers, during the performance of a simple motor task with their dominant hand, MS patients showed increased activation of several areas of the sensorimotor network, including the ipsilateral SMA, the ipsilateral superior frontal sulcus, and the contralateral thalamus. The increased recruitment of the SMA was correlated with the peak height and position of the mean diffusivity (MD) histogram of the normal-appearing grey matter (NAGM). In contrast, when compared to MS patients, healthy subjects showed increased activation of the ipsilateral primary SMC. When the results obtained from the analysis of the two tasks (with the dominant and the nondominant hand) were combined, MS patients showed increased activation of the SMA and reduced activation of the ipsilateral SMC. The most probable explanation of these findings might be enhanced "transcallosal inhibition," a mechanism that has been postulated to be responsible for the control of homologous hand muscle during unilateral movements [39]. The role of the corpus callosum in interhemispheric connectivity, and of subtle NABT damage in eliciting functional cortical changes, has been underpinned by two other fMRI studies [40, 41]. By measuring low-frequency BOLD fluctuations, a reduced functional connectivity was shown between the right and the left hemisphere primary motor cortices in MS patients [40]. Strong correlations between MD histogram peak height of the normal-appearing white matter (NAWM) and the extent of displacement of the SMA have been shown in patients with migraine and nonspecific T2-weighted abnormalities [41].

Rocca et al. [42] assessed the brain pattern of cortical activations in patients with SPMS during the performance of simple motor tasks and investigated whether the extent of cortical brain activations correlated with the extent of brain structural changes. Compared to healthy volunteers, SPMS patients showed more significant activations of several regions located in the frontal and parietal lobes. Strong correlations were found between relative activations of cortical areas of the motor network and the severity of structural changes of the NAWM and NAGM, suggesting that cortical plasticity might have a role in limiting the clinical impact of MS-related damage.

Preliminary work has shown that the pattern of movement-associated cortical activations in RRMS is determined by both the extent of brain injury and disability [43]. Cortical activations during a simple motor task have been studied in three groups of RRMS patients classified as follows: group 1, no clinical impairment and normal "axonal equivalents"; group 2, no clinical impairment and 20% reduction in "axonal equivalents"; and group 3, 40% reduction in the movement performance of the hand and 20% reduction in "axonal equivalents". The "injury contrast" (i.e., group 2 vs group 1) showed increased activation of the SMA and premotor cortex in patients of group 2, whereas the "impairment contrast" (group 3 vs group 2) showed increased activation of the SMC and of the parietal cortex, bilaterally, in patients of group 3.

The results of all these studies suggest that there might be a "natural history" of the functional reorganization of the cerebral cortex in MS patients, which might be characterized at the beginning of the disease by increased recruitment of those areas "normally" devoted to the performance of a given task, such as the primary SMC and the SMA in case of a motor task. At a later stage, bilateral activation of these regions is seen first, followed by widespread recruitment of additional areas, which are usually recruited in normal people to perform novel or complex tasks. This notion has been supported by the results of a recent study [44], which has provided a direct demonstration that, during the performance of a simple motor task, MS patients activate some regions that are part of a frontoparietal circuit whose activation in healthy subjects typically occurs during object manipulation [44].

Increased recruitment of several cortical areas has been found in RRMS patients during the performance of tasks designed to explore sustained attention [45-48] and memory [48-50]. During these tasks, fMRI activity is greater in patients with better cognitive function than in those with lower cognitive function [47, 48]. The correlations found by some of these authors between the extent of activation in specific brain regions during the performance of different cognitive tasks, brain T_2 lesion load [48], and brain parenchymal volume [46] suggest that these functional changes might represent adaptive mechanisms to the underlying structural pathology.

fMRI in Patients with Primary Progressive MS

Patients with primary progressive (PP) MS are characterized by progressive accumulation of disability from the onset of the disease [51] despite the small amount of lesions visible on conventional MRI scans of the brain and cord [52]. However, several quantitative MRI techniques have shown diffuse NABT changes in brain and cervical cord in these patients [52]. Work with DTI has also detected widespread cortical grey matter pathology [9].

At present, only two studies [53, 54] have investigated the role of cortical plasticity in limiting the functional consequences of widespread tissue damage in patients with PPMS. In one study [53], the patterns of brain activations following simple and complex motor tasks were assessed in PPMS patients with variable degrees of motor impairment and in sex- and age-matched controls. Significant cortical activation changes during the performance of both the simple and the complex motor tasks were found in PPMS patients, who showed different patterns of cortical activation with their varying degrees of clinical impairment. During the performance of a simple motor task with the clinically unaffected limbs, PPMS patients had more significant activations of the contralateral SMA, the SII bilaterally, and several regions of the frontal and temporal (insula and superior temporal gyrus) lobes in comparison with healthy volunteers. These findings indicate a marked cortical reorganization taking place in brain regions involved in different phases of movement planning and execution. Interestingly, the observed pattern of cortical activations involved a widespread network usually considered to function in motor, sensory, and multimodal integration processing [55]. During the performance of a simple task with an affected limb, PPMS patients showed increased activations of the ipsilateral CMA and postcentral gyrus. Since CMA activation in healthy subjects has been related to learning of new motor tasks and is also thought to reflect task difficulty [56, 57], a possible explanation for the increased CMA recruitment found in PPMS patients might be that the patients tended to perceive the simple experimental task as a sort of novel task, which consequently needed to be "re-learned." Finally, during the execution of a more complex task, PPMS patients showed increased activation of the ipsilateral thalamus, the MFG, bilaterally, and several other sensory regions, including an ipsilateral area located in the visual cortex. Visual-sensory interactions are known to occur in humans [58], and, again, they might be enhanced in PPMS patients in an attempt to compensate for the functional impairment secondary to subcortical white matter damage.

In another study [54], the extent of brain activations during simple hand movements was correlated to lesion burden as seen on T_2-weighted MRI scans, MT ratio and average MD of brain T_2-visible lesions, NABT, and cervical cord from PPMS patients with a fully normal motor function of their right upper limbs. The tested hypothesis was that if cortical adaptive responses have the potential to limit the accumulation of disability in patients with PPMS after tissue injury, the extent of such changes should be greater with increasing MS-related pathology. Consistently with this hypothesis, strong correlations between the extent of the fMRI activations of several sensorimotor areas and several MR metrics of structural damage of the brain and the cervical cord were found. These findings suggest that not only brain, but also cord pathology can induce cortical changes with the potential to limit the functional impact of the disease. To assess the role of cervical cord pathology in isolation in eliciting brain functional reorganization, movement-associated cortical activation has been recently investigated in patients with a previous episode of isolated acute myelitis of probably demyelinating origin and lack of brain damage [59] and in patients with Devic's neuromyelitis optica [60]. In both these studies, the relationship between the extent of cortical reorganization and the extent of cord pathology, measured using MTI, was also evaluated. Compared to healthy volunteers, patients with myelitis had increased recruitment of several areas mainly located in the ipsilateral hemisphere [59, 60]. Several strong correlations were found between the extent of fMRI activations and MTI metrics of cervical cord damage [59, 60].

Conclusion

fMRI has the potential to provide important information about cortical reorganization following MS tissue damage which should improve our understanding of the factors associated with the accumulation of irreversible disability in MS. Although the role of cortical reorganization in limiting the functional impact of structural damage in MS is still not definitively proved, the available data support the concept that cortical adaptive responses may have an important role in compensating for MS irreversible tissue damage, such as axonal loss. As suggested by a study of a patient with an early diagnosis of subacute combined degeneration, demyelination alone is in fact unlikely to lead to overt functional cortical changes [61]. In conclusion, the presently available fMRI data suggest that the rate of accumulation of disability in MS may be a function not only of tissue loss, but also of the progressive failure of the adaptive capacity of the cortex. Enhancing any beneficial effects of this cortical adaptive plasticity should be considered a potential target for therapy of the disease.

References

1. Filippi M, Grossman RI (2002) MRI techniques to monitor MS evolution: the present and the future [review]. Neurology 58:1147-1153
2. Ferguson B, Matyszak MK, Esiri MM, Perry VH (1997) Axonal damage in acute multiple sclerosis lesions. Brain 120:393-399
3. Trapp BD, Ransohoff R, Rudick R (1999) Axonal pathology in multiple sclerosis: relationship to neurologic disability. Curr Opin Neurol 12:295-302
4. Kidd D, Barkhof F, McConnel R et al (1999) Cortical lesions in multiple sclerosis. Brain 122:17-26
5. Brownell B, Hughes JT (1962) The distribution of plaques in the cerebrum in multiple sclerosis. J Neurol Neurosurg Psychiatry 25:315-320
6. Peterson JW, Bö L, Mork S et al (2001) Transected neurites, apoptotic neurons, and reduced inflammation in cortical multiple sclerosis lesions. Ann Neurol 50:389-400
7. Ge Y, Grossman RI, Udupa JK et al (2002) Magnetization transfer ratio histogram analysis of normal-appearing grey matter and normal-appearing white matter in multiple sclerosis. J Comput Assist Tomogr 26:62-68
8. Cercignani M, Bozzali M, Iannucci G et al (2001) Magnetisation transfer ratio and mean diffusivity of normal appearing white and grey matter from patients with multiple sclerosis. J Neurol Neurosurg Psychiatry 70:311-317
9. Bozzali M, Cercignani M, Sormani MP et al (2002) Quantification of brain grey matter damage in different MS phenotypes by use of diffusion tensor MR imaging. AJNR Am J Neuroradiol 23:985-988
10. Sarchielli P, Presciutti O, Tarducci R et al (2002) Localized (1)H magnetic resonance spectroscopy in mainly cortical grey matter of patients with multiple sclerosis. J Neurol 249:902-910
11. Ogawa S, Menon RS, Kim SG, Ugurbil K (1998) On the characteristics of functional magnetic resonance imaging of the brain [review]. Annu Rev Biophys Biomol Struct 27:447-474
12. Vanzetta I, Grinvald A (1999) Increased cortical oxidative metabolism due to sensory stimulation: implications for functional brain imaging. Science 286:1555-1558
13. Bandettini PA, Jesmanowicz A, Wong EC, Hyde JS (1993) Processing strategies for time-course data sets in functional MRI of the human brain. Magn Reson Med 30:161-173
14. Worsley KJ, Friston KJ (1995) Analysis of fMRI time-series revisited – again. Neuroimage 2:173-181

15. Clanet M, Berry I, Boulanouar K (1997) Functional imaging in multiple sclerosis. Int MS J 4:26-32
16. Lee M, Reddy H, Johansen-Berg H et al (2000) The motor cortex shows adaptive functional changes to brain injury from multiple sclerosis. Ann Neurol 47:606-613
17. Werring DJ, Bullmore ET, Toosy AT et al (2000) Recovery from optic neuritis is associated with a change in the distribution of cerebral response to visual stimulation: a functional magnetic resonance imaging study. J Neurol Neurosurg Psychiatry 68:441-449
18. Reddy H, Narayanan S, Matthews PM et al (2000) Relating axonal injury to functional recovery in MS. Neurology 54:236-239
19. Rombouts SA, Lazeron RH, Scheltens P et al (1998) Visual activation patterns in patients with optic neuritis: an fMRI pilot study. Neurology 50:1896-1899
20. Langkilde AR, Frederiksen JL, Rostrup E, Larsson HB (2002) Functional MRI of the visual cortex and visual testing in patients with previous optic neuritis Eur J Neurol 9:277-286
21. Reddy H, Narayanan S, Arnoutelis R et al (2000) Evidence for adaptive functional changes in the cerebral cortex with axonal injury from multiple sclerosis. Brain 123:2314-2320
22. Noseworthy JH, Lucchinetti C, Rodriguez M, Weinshenker BG (2000) Multiple sclerosis. N Engl J Med 343:938-952
23. Iannucci G, Tortorella C, Rovaris M et al (2000) Prognostic value of MR and magnetization transfer imaging findings in patients with clinically isolated syndromes suggestive of multiple sclerosis at presentation. AJNR Am J Neuroradiol 21:1034-1038
24. Brex PA, Jenkins R, Fox NC et al (2000) Detection of ventricular enlargement in patients at the earliest clinical stage of MS. Neurology 54:1689-1691
25. Filippi M, Inglese M, Rovaris M et al (2000) Magnetization transfer imaging to monitor the evolution of MS: a 1-year follow-up study. Neurology 55:940-946
26. Chard DT, Griffin CM, Parker GJ et al (2000) Brain atrophy in clinically early relapsing-remitting multiple sclerosis. Brain 125:327-337
27. Kapeller P, McLean MA, Griffin CM et al (2001) Preliminary evidence for neuronal damage in cortical grey matter and normal appearing white matter in short duration relapsing-remitting multiple sclerosis: a quantitative MR spectroscopic imaging study. J Neurol 248:131-138
28. Toosy AT, Werring DJ, Bullmore ET et al (2002) Functional magnetic resonance imaging of the cortical response to photic stimulation in humans following optic neuritis recovery. Neurosci Lett 330:255-259
29. Russ MO, Cleff U, Lanfermann H et al (2002) Functional magnetic resonance imaging in acute unilateral optic neuritis. J Neuroimaging 12:339-350
30. Rocca MA, Mezzapesa DM, Falini A et al (2003) Evidence for axonal pathology and adaptive cortical reorganisation in patients at presentation with clinically isolated syndromes suggestive of MS. Neuroimage 18:847-855
31. Filippi M, Rocca MA, Mezzapesa DM et al (2004) Simple and complex movement-associated functional MRI changes in patients at presentation with clinically isolated syndromes suggestive of multiple sclerosis. Hum Brain Mapp 21:108-117
32. Pantano P, Iannetti GD, Caramia F et al (2002) Cortical motor reorganization after a single clinical attack of multiple sclerosis. Brain 125:1607-1615
33. Pantano P, Mainero C, Iannetti GD et al (2002) Contribution of corticospinal tract damage to cortical motor reorganization after a single clinical attack of multiple sclerosis. Neuroimage 17:1837-1843
34. McDonald WI, Compston A, Edan G et al (2001) Recommended diagnostic criteria for multiple sclerosis: guidelines from the International Panel on the Diagnosis of Multiple Sclerosis. Ann Neurol 50:121-127
35. Rocca MA, Falini A, Colombo B et al (2002) Adaptive functional changes in the cere-

bral cortex of patients with nondisabling multiple sclerosis correlate with the extent of brain structural damage. Ann Neurol 51:330-339
36. Filippi M, Rocca MA, Colombo B et al (2002) Functional magnetic resonance imaging correlates of fatigue in multiple sclerosis. Neuroimage 15:559-567
37. Filippi M, Rocca MA, Minicucci L et al (1999) Magnetization transfer imaging of patients with definite MS and negative conventional MRI. Neurology 52:845-848
38. Rocca MA, Pagani E, Ghezzi A et al (2003) Functional cortical changes in patients with MS and non-specific conventional MRI scans of the brain. Neuroimage 19:826-836
39. Liepert J, Dettmers C, Terborg C, Weiller C (2001) Inhibition of ipsilateral motor cortex during phasic generation of low force. Clin Neurophysiol 112:114-121
40. Lowe MJ, Phillips MD, Lurito JT et al (2002) Multiple sclerosis: low-frequency temporal blood oxygen level-dependent fluctuations indicate reduced functional connectivity initial results. Radiology 224:184-192
41. Rocca MA, Colombo B, Pagani E et al (2003) Evidence for cortical functional changes in patients with migraine and white matter abnormalities on conventional and diffusion tensor MRI. Stroke 34:665-670
42. Rocca MA, Gavazzi C, Mezzapesa DM et al (2003) A functional magnetic resonance imaging study of patients with secondary progressive multiple sclerosis. Neuroimage 19:1770-1777
43. Reddy H, Narayanan S, Mitsumori T et al (2002) Functional brain reorganization for hand movement in patients with multiple sclerosis: defining distinct effects of injury and disability. Brain 125: 2646-2657
44. Filippi M, Rocca MA, Mezzapesa DM et al (2004) A functional MRI study of cortical activations associated with object manipulation in patients with MS. Neuroimage 21:1147-1154
45. Staffen W, Mair A, Zauner H et al (2002) Cognitive function and fMRI in patients with multiple sclerosis: evidence for compensatory cortical activation during an attention task. Brain 125:1275-1282
46. Parry AM, Scott RB, Palace J et al (2003) Potentially adaptive functional changes in cognitive processing for patients with multiple sclerosis and their acute modulation by rivastigmine. Brain 126:2750-2760
47. Penner IK, Rausch M, Kappos L et al (2003) Analysis of impairment related functional architecture in MS patients during performance of different attention tasks. J Neurol 250:461-472
48. Mainero C, Caramia F, Pozzilli C et al (2004) fMRI evidence of brain reorganization during attention and memory tasks in multiple sclerosis. Neuroimage 21:858-867
49. Hillary FG, Chiaravalloti ND, Ricker JH et al (2003) An investigation of working memory rehearsal in multiple sclerosis using fMRI. J Clin Exp Neuropsychol 25:965-978
50. Wishart HA, Saykin AJ, McDonald BC et al (2004) Brain activation patterns associated with working memory in relapsing-remitting MS. Neurology 62:234-238
51. Thompson AJ, Montalban X, Barkhof F et al (2000) Diagnostic criteria for primary progressive multiple sclerosis: a position paper. Ann Neurol 47:831-835
52. Filippi M, Comi G (2002) Primary progressive multiple sclerosis. Springer, Milan Heidelberg New York
53. Rocca MA, Matthews PM, Caputo D et al (2002) Evidence for widespread movement-associated functional MRI changes in patients with PPMS. Neurology 58:866-872
54. Filippi M, Rocca MA, Falini A et al (2002) Correlations between structural CNS damage and functional MRI changes in primary progressive MS. Neuroimage 15:537-546
55. Mesulam MM (1998) From sensation to cognition. Brain 121:1013-1052
56. Rao SM, Binder JR, Bandettini PA et al (1993) Functional magnetic resonance imaging of complex human movements. Neurology 43:2311-2318

57. Paus T, Petrides M, Evans AC, Meyer E (1993) Role of the human anterior cingulate cortex in the control of oculomotor, manual, and speech responses: a positron emission tomography study. J Neurophysiol 70:453-469
58. de Gelder B (2000) Neuroscience. More to seeing than meets the eye. Science 289:1148-1149
59. Rocca MA, Mezzapesa DM, Ghezzi A et al (2003) Cord damage elicits brain functional reorganization after a single episode of myelitis. Neurology 61:1078-1085
60. Rocca MA, Agosta F, Mezzapesa DM et al (2004) A functional MRI study of movement-associated cortical changes in patients with Devic's neuromyelitis optica. Neuroimage 21:1061-1068
61. Filippi M, Rocca MA, Rossi P et al (2003) Demyelination and cortical reorganization: functional MRI data from a case of subacute combined degeneration. Neuroimage 18:558-563

Subject Index

GPSR Compliance
The European Union's (EU) General Product Safety Regulation (GPSR) is a set of rules that requires consumer products to be safe and our obligations to ensure this.

If you have any concerns about our products, you can contact us on

ProductSafety@springernature.com

In case Publisher is established outside the EU, the EU authorized representative is:

Springer Nature Customer Service Center GmbH
Europaplatz 3
69115 Heidelberg, Germany

www.ingramcontent.com/pod-product-compliance
Lightning Source LLC
Chambersburg PA
CBHW071342230926
51846CB00002B/423
9788847021754